PROTECT YOUR PREGNANCY

Bonnie C. Campos
RN-C, MS

Jennifer Brown

[handwritten inscription: Joan & Richard, Thanks for all your interest and support. Jennifer Brown]

McGraw-Hill

New York   Chicago   San Francisco   Lisbon   London
Madrid   Mexico City   Milan   New Delhi   San Juan
Seoul   Singapore   Sydney   Toronto

1 2 3 4 5 6 7 8 9 0   DOC / DOC   0 9 8 7 6 5 4 3

ISBN 0-07-140874-6

McGraw-Hill books are available at special discounts to use as premiums and sales promotions, or for use in corporate training programs. For more information, please write to the Director of Special Sales, Professional Publishing, McGraw-Hill, Two Penn Plaza, New York, NY 10121-2298. Or contact your local bookstore.

The purpose of this book is to educate. It is sold with the understanding that the author and publisher shall have neither liability nor responsibility for any injury caused or alleged to be caused directly or indirectly by the information in this book. While every effort has been made to ensure the book's accuracy, its contents should not be construed as medical advice. Each person's health needs are unique. To obtain recommendations appropriate to your particular situation, please consult a qualified health care professional.

 This book is printed on recycled, acid-free paper containing a minimum of 50% recycled de-inked paper.

Library of Congress Cataloging-in-Publication Data

Campos, Bonnie.
  Protect your pregnancy / Bonnie Campos and Jennifer C. Brown.
    p. cm.
  ISBN 0-07-140874-6 (pbk. : alk. paper)
    1. Pregnancy—Popular works. 2. Pregnancy—Complications—Popular
works. I. Brown, Jennifer C. II. Title.
  RG525.C318 2004
  618.2'4—dc22

2003024121

Acknowledgments

We would like to thank a great many people for their interest, support, and expertise during the writing of this book. Marjory Ruderman supplied public health information, and, along with Dani James and Gail Gugel, read early drafts of the proposal and chapters of the book. Pete Mondale gave us feedback and advice on research methodology. Mickey Parel, CNM, introduced us to hypnobirthing. Doula Susan Lucas gave us insights into how doulas can help during labor. Fitness coach Marian Lally explained the purpose and importance of exercise during pregnancy. Dr. Benjamin Purow, MD, explained medical terminology. Members of the Maternity Center, Bethesda, Maryland, and Birthcare and Women's Health of Virginia, particularly director Marsha Jackson, CNM, described how midwives work. Marilyn Baker, CNM, read drafts of chapters and offered much enthusiasm and support. Julie Sorenson, physician assistant at Simmonds and Simmonds, an ob-gyn practice, clarified how doctors and midwives work together. Paul E. Lewis, MD, shared his wealth of knowledge regarding obstetrical care. Ann Jordan, RNC, and Paula McNinch, CNP, read chapters of the book and updated our information. The perinatal nurses of the Kaiser TLC Program, who dedicate their lives to caring for expectant mothers and their families, reassured us that the information in this book will benefit women who are seeking pregnancy or expecting a baby. Many women contributed stories of their pregnancies and children's births. Some vestiges of these stories made it into the book and many did not, but all confirmed to us that pregnancies and births occur in a staggering variety of ways. We could not have written this book without the writing expertise and editing advice of Jennifer's father, Fred Brown. We are also indebted to our editor, Nancy Hancock, who had a clear vision for what this book would be and kept us on track. Nancy's assistant, Meg Leder, helped us through the steps of creating this book with unflappable calm. Much gratitude is also extended to our agent, Mary Tahan, of Clausen, Mays, and Tahan, for her guidance, warmth, and patience.

Also from Bonnie:
I would like to thank my husband Jim, for his unfailing love, encouragement, and understanding that kept me anchored to the importance of this book. Thanks to mydaughters Martina and Nina, and my son Orlando, for their patience andacceptance that I was busy "writing" and who encouraged me to keep going, and to my sister Connie, the best listener, who offered support and love when I was out of "steam."

Also from Jenny:
I want to give a special thanks to my husband Chris, for timely nudges, no-nonsense advice, a willing ear, companionship, mutual admiration, and love.

---

*I dedicate this book to all the women who want
to help themselves have a healthy baby.
And to my parents, Marie and Chris Campos,
who taught me that dreams start with action.*
—B.C. Campos

*This book is dedicated to my parents,
Frederick and Sara E. Brown,
ever seekers of truth and beauty,
and to my grandmother, Anna H. Erickson.*
—J.C. Brown

Contents

1

Planning Your Pregnancy Journey

 Sonia's Journal

> *Dear Journal,*
>
> *I can't believe it! I'm pregnant! I'm going to have a baby! Me, a mother. It's unbelievable! I returned the call from Dr. Joseph's office. The nurse said, "Congratulations, you're pregnant!" I couldn't breathe. Can it be real? We've been trying so long. I've made my first prenatal appointment and I need to get some lab tests done. And I'll need some more information from Brian and my parents to be able to fill out the medical history forms. I think that's all. I could barely hear any of it my heart was pounding so hard. I'm going to write down everything that happens during this pregnancy and all of my feelings about it.*

You are thinking about having a baby. You feel ready, but you want to learn everything you can before plunging in.

In fact, your instincts are good. The more knowledge you have about pregnancy, the better time you'll have along the way.

Imagine you're about to plan a trip around the world, a trip that will take slightly less than a year and require a significant amount of time and money. You'd probably want to learn everything you could about where you were going and the best way to get there. Knowledge and careful planning are critical elements to a successful journey, so you'd want to know how to prepare your mind and body.

That's the intent of this book: to guide you and your partner through your incredibly exciting journey of pregnancy and birth. To that end, we'll provide straightforward, reassuring answers to your questions about how to safeguard your pregnancy and the birth of your baby.

Mental Preparation

The first step in having a baby is examining your current situation with your partner and then taking a look at how your life might change with pregnancy. The following exercise may help both of you clarify your feelings about having a baby. Don't be afraid if you find that your opinions differ. It's better to know about these differences early on so you can talk them through.

We suggest that you and your partner write down the questions below and answer them separately. Share your answers at a time when you can both pay full attention to each other.

These are suggested questions; that is, you can tailor them to your specific situation. Remind each other that this is how you believe you'll be, and that no one can predict exactly how things will turn out. (Even if you're already pregnant, you may still find answering most of the following questions helpful.)

1. What do I see as the obstacles to having a baby?
2. How can I overcome these barriers?
3. Do I believe my relationship can handle the work of planning a pregnancy, nine months of being pregnant, and providing care for a child through years of dependency?
4. Do I have any idea what kind of parent my partner will be?
5. Do I have any idea what kind of parent I will be?
6. Can I contribute a great deal of time and money to a new member of the family, and am I willing to do it?
7. Who will have primary responsibility to care for the baby? Will it be equal?
8. Who will make major decisions for the baby? Will it be equal?
9. How will being a parent impact my job/career?
10. How will being a parent impact my partner's job/career?

11. Do I feel my partner and I can continue with our current work schedules? If not, who should change, and why?
12. How will being a parent impact my social life—vacations, weekends, free time?
13. How will being a parent impact my partner's social life—vacations, weekends, free time?
14. If I decide not to get pregnant now, will my biological clock allow me to plan for a baby later?

Discuss how you think you should address any differences in your answers. Then ask yourselves if you feel you can move forward to plan this journey together?

Parenting is not for everyone. If you find you have major disagreements about becoming a parent, now is the time to recognize it and to develop a plan to resolve the differences or admit to yourself (and your partner) that you're not ready to take the journey. Communication is crucial in a relationship, especially when planning a family. In some situations, you as a couple may want to consider getting counseling to assist with resolving your differences or establishing better communication.

Physical Preparation

Pregnancy is not just a physical event—it's a journey. And before embarking on any journey, any adventure, you should feel your best, so you can savor every moment of a totally new experience. Imagine planning a two-week hike along the Appalachian trail and not having exercised in months. You may have just put in weeks of long hours at work to finish a project on time, subsisting on carry-out meals from the nearest fast food place. It's more likely that when the grueling job was finally completed, you'd want to sleep for the first few days rather than embarking upon a physical and emotional adventure. In the same manner, you need to be physically fit for a pregnancy journey.

Most women know it's important to be healthy when contemplating a pregnancy. But how do you know if you are healthy? What things should you change, increase, decrease, start up, stop, or have checked out? Is it important to be in peak physical condition? What is that like? How can you get into great physical condition?

These questions and more may be running through your mind. The next few pages will offer suggestions for what areas to look at in preparation for becoming pregnant. Keep in mind that any positive changes toward a healthy body and mind will have a positive impact on you and your baby. After all, your goal is to have a happier, healthier pregnancy and baby.

In fact, this is a good way to start: by telling yourself that you want to have a healthy baby and a happy pregnancy experience. This begins the process of cultivating a positive attitude. Next, you can ask yourself, "Am I healthy and do I have healthy lifestyle habits?" And if not: "How can I improve or change, in order to be healthier?" Don't forget to ask your partner if he feels he has lifestyle habits that need improving. You're in this adventure together, and some lifestyle changes will have a beneficial impact on the whole family's health. Changing a lifestyle habit is much easier when you're not pregnant!

Changing Unhealthy Habits

Lifestyle habits that are *not healthy* include smoking, using alcohol or other drugs, overeating and undereating, and not taking steps to alleviate stress. If you feel you have some unhealthy habits, the first thing for you to understand is that you don't have to go it alone. There are resources available to help you change.

Smoking and Pregnancy

By now, everyone knows the dangers of smoking. Health problems from smoking can occur even if you don't smoke but live or work around someone who does. What you might not know is that smoking affects women differently than men. It can alter hormone levels, which in turn can affect fertility, cause miscarriages, and lead to early menopause. Smoking can interfere with your baby's use of vitamin B, which is necessary for normal harmone production.

Smoking has a dramatically dangerous effect on the fetus. When a pregnant woman inhales cigarette smoke, the carbon monoxide in cigarettes decreases the oxygen in her blood. Therefore, there is less oxygen getting to the baby, oxygen that's vital to the baby's development. Babies born to women who smoke may have respiratory problems, sleep problems, learning disorders, and are generally smaller in size. And being smaller in stature and weight can mean an increased susceptibility to diseases and even to death.

Getting Help with Quitting

We know that to stop smoking is not easy. But you can do it. Wanting to be pregnant and have a healthy baby should be an extra incentive. Get help from others if your own efforts fail. Ask former smokers what worked for them, and get information from health care providers. Talk with your doctor about steps to help you quit or decrease your smoking before you're pregnant. Make it your goal to have stopped smoking at least three months before trying to conceive.

If you're unable to quit beforehand, it's important to realize that at least cutting down on smoking during the pregnancy—or better, stopping altogether—can still be beneficial. Any decrease in the amount of smoke in your lungs may mean more oxygen can get to your baby.

Here are some suggestions to try if you're *not* pregnant. Try talking to your doctor about:

- A smoking cessation class.
- A prescription for the nicotine patch, which contains time-released nicotine transferred through your skin. This specifically should *not* be used during pregnancy. The patch will maintain the amount of nicotine your body craves without the smoke and other toxins.
- A medication often used as an antidepressant is thought to decrease the craving for nicotine (also specifically not to be used during pregnancy).

Alcohol and Drugs

You may enjoy a glass of wine with dinner or a beer at the end of the workday or at the end of a busy week. You may even smoke marijuana occasionally. You may be wondering how harmful these habits are. The answer is: If you are contemplating having a baby, *any amount* of alcohol or illicit drug is not advisable because they can impact a pregnancy dramatically. Studies have shown that the heavy use of alcohol or occasional bingeing may cause developmental problems in a fetus's major organs. And as well as adversely affecting your baby's health, the use of drugs can affect the way your body handles pregnancy and your ability to care for your baby.

Getting Help with Quitting

The most important time to stop use of alcohol or drugs is before you try to conceive. And then you should plan to abstain from these chemicals throughout your pregnancy. It may be hard to stop completely. Giving up a habit you've had for some time may cause you some stress. But the stress of pregnancy may make it even more difficult to stop these habits. As with smoking, it's easier to handle the stress of quitting before you're pregnant. Ask your partner to join you in abstaining so you can support each other. Remind yourself repeatedly that by giving up drugs or alcohol during your pregnancy, you're doing everything you can to have a healthy baby.

In your effort to stop taking drugs or alcohol, you may discover you have an addiction. In fact, addiction to illicit drugs or alcohol is an illness and will require specific medical treatment by a specialist. If you suspect you may have an addiction problem, get help from your health care provider.

THOUGHT TO REMEMBER
Whatever you do when you're pregnant, your baby also does! Try to picture your baby having a small glass of wine with dinner or a cigarette with coffee!

Pregnancy with a Chronic Medical Condition

Many women with chronic (or long-term) illnesses or medical conditions are successfully undertaking pregnancy and birth. In most cases the desire to have a baby is reasonable and you can expect to have a healthy pregnancy. However, in your pregnancy planning, you should make time to work with your doctor to be sure the chronic condition is under control and that any medications you need to take will not interfere with producing a healthy baby. Indeed, many health problems are treated with some kind of medication. Sometimes these drugs may be harmful during pregnancy. On the other hand, going without a prescribed medication may be harmful to you. Having a medical condition that requires medication that may not be taken during pregnancy does not mean you cannot become pregnant. Your doctor may be able to change your prescription to a medication you can use during pregnancy.

Some of the more common chronic conditions that need to be under control before starting a pregnancy are asthma, diabetes, hypertension, heart and lung diseases, blood disorders (sickle cell anemia), some cancers, bacterial infections, depression and bipolar disorder, epilepsy (or other seizure disorders), severe allergies, and autoimmune diseases like lupus.

If you hope to become pregnant and you have a chronic medical condition or take medication on a regular basis, you should consult with your OB/GYN provider. He or she may consult with the doctor who diagnosed your problem and/or continues to treat you. Together they can determine whether a plan can be developed to give you medication that will be effective for your condition and yet is not harmful to your baby. Occasionally your OB provider may refer you to a perinatologist—a high-risk obstetrics specialist—to evaluate how your condition could be affected by the pregnancy.

Medication Labeling

Even without a chronic medical condition, you may rely on prescription or over-the-counter medications to alleviate occasional illnesses or health problems. When planning a pregnancy, it is important to review the medications you take either regularly or occasionally to be sure they're not harmful to your pregnancy.

While some medications are known to be harmful to fetuses, the effects from others are unknown. In some cases, no tests have been done to determine the effects on pregnant women, or reports on women taking the medication have not been collected and analyzed.

In the face of uncertainty, many physicians have their patients only take medications that are known to be relatively safe.

The FDA (Food and Drug Administration) has developed a system for classifying medications according to their known or unknown effects on a pregnancy or the unborn baby. Medications that can cause developmental problems in the unborn child are called *teratologens*. The current FDA medication classification system rates drugs A, B, C, D, or X. One of these classifications can be found on each of the medications you take.

FDA Drug Category

A   Adequate, well-controlled studies in pregnant women have not shown an increased risk of fetal abnormalities.

B   Animal studies have revealed no evidence of harm to the fetus, however, there are no adequate and well-controlled studies in pregnant women.
Or:
Animal studies have shown an adverse effect, but adequate and well-controlled studies in pregnant women have failed to demonstrate risk to the fetus.

C   Animal studies have shown an adverse effect and there are no adequate and well-controlled studies in pregnant women.
Or:
No animal studies have been conducted and there are no adequate and well-controlled studies in pregnant women.

D   Studies, adequate, well-controlled or observational, in pregnant women have demonstrated a risk to the fetus. However, the benefits of therapy may outweigh the potential risk.

X   Studies, adequate, well-controlled or observational, in animals or pregnant women have demonstrated positive evidence of fetal abnormalities. The use of the product is contraindicated in women who may become pregnant.

(From the U.S. Food and Drug Administration (FDA). See fda.gov/fdac/ features/2001/301_preg.html.)

The FDA is planning to improve the current rating system by including more specific information on a medication's effect on fertility, pregnancy, and breast-feeding. By knowing more about the medications you take, you and your doctor will be better able to weigh the benefits and risks of continuing a medication during your pregnancy. To be certain of what medications, herbs, and over-the-counter medicine you can use, speak to your doctor before you take them.

Weight Control Before Pregnancy

If You're Overweight

Ideally, you should be at a good weight when you start a pregnancy. Remember, pregnancy is a physical event. A great deal will be asked of your body. But you may have problems getting pregnant if your weight is excessive. Being overweight can make your body work harder and tire faster because excess weight is a physical stress. And once you're pregnant, significant weight gain can affect how well you do in labor and even impact your baby's health.

If you're overweight before pregnancy, it may be difficult to shed the pounds gained in pregnancy after having your baby. And the psychological impact of continuing to be overweight can alter your self-esteem and your outlook on life in general.

We're not naïve: Losing weight is very difficult for many women. You may need some expert help. Your doctor can determine whether you have a medical condition that is causing you to gain weight and requires medical intervention. He or she can also provide referrals to professionals who can help you with implementing an exercise routine, getting proper nutrition, and altering eating habits. A nutritionist can assist you with a safe weight-loss program that is geared to your becoming pregnant. By asking for professional help, you will have the tools and support to successfully attain your ideal weight and level of fitness.

If You're Underweight

Being *underweight* may alter the levels of your reproductive hormones, and you may therefore have difficulty becoming pregnant. If you do become pregnant, being underweight during pregnancy may mean that your baby may be undernourished.

To increase your weight to a normal level, your doctor can put you on a nutritious diet to boost your intake of calories or investigate possible causes for your inability to attain a normal weight. Your problem may be easily resolved once you pay more attention to what you're eating and stick with a healthy diet. Try following the USDA's food guiding pyramid found in Chapter 3 to help you gain weight in a healthy manner.

Your Ideal Weight at Pregnancy

To find out if you're at a good weight to attempt pregnancy, calculate your body mass index (BMI). In Table 1–1, find your height in the left column. Read across the row horizontally until you find your weight. Look at the number in bold above where you stopped at your weight. That number is your body mass index. If it's between 20 and 25, you're at a normal weight. If it's above or below, you are overweight or underweight. For example, if your height is 5 feet 3 inches, or 63 inches, and your weight is 118 pounds, your body mass index number is 21. Since this is between 20 and 25, you're at a good weight.

The number you find is your BMI. Compare your BMI to the following weight ranges:

Underweight: < 18.5
Healthful weight: 18.5–24.9
Overweight: 25.0–29.9
Obese: 30 and over

Exercising Before Pregnancy

Prior to pregnancy is a good time to create lifelong good health habits. And regular exercise is a good habit. If you already exercise regularly, continue your program. If you aren't exercising at least three times a

TABLE 1-1. BODY MASS INDEX CHART*														
	BMI													
	19	**20**	**21**	**22**	**23**	**24**	**25**	**26**	**27**	**28**	**29**	**30**	**31**	**32**
Height (inches)						Weight (pounds)								
58	91	96	100	105	110	115	119	124	129	134	138	143	148	153
59	94	99	104	109	114	119	124	128	133	138	143	148	153	158
60	97	102	107	112	118	123	128	133	138	143	148	153	158	163
61	100	106	111	116	122	127	132	137	143	148	153	158	164	169
62	104	109	115	120	126	131	136	142	147	153	158	164	169	175
63	107	113	118	124	130	135	141	146	152	158	163	169	175	180
64	110	116	122	128	134	140	145	151	157	163	169	174	180	186
65	114	120	126	132	138	144	150	156	162	168	174	180	186	192
66	118	124	130	136	142	148	155	161	167	173	179	186	192	198
67	121	127	134	140	146	153	159	166	172	178	185	191	198	204
68	125	131	138	144	151	158	164	171	177	184	190	197	203	210
69	128	135	142	149	155	162	169	176	182	189	196	203	209	216
70	132	139	146	153	160	167	174	181	188	195	202	209	216	222
71	136	143	150	157	165	172	179	186	193	200	208	215	222	229
72	140	147	154	162	169	177	184	191	199	206	213	221	228	235
73	144	151	159	166	174	182	1891	197	204	212	219	227	235	242
74	148	155	163	171	179	186	94	202	210	218	225	233	241	249

*Source: National Heart and Lung Institute.

week, you should increase your activity slowly, but try to start doing something.

Most OB providers will urge you to undertake some kind of moderate exercise on a regular basis during your pregnancy. But if you wait until you're pregnant, you may feel overwhelmed at starting something that may make you perspire and be out of breath or off balance. Try to choose an activity that you will want to and be able to continue after you're pregnant, such as walking, swimming, or yoga. Walking 20 minutes every other day is a safe way to start. If you can afford it, join a health club and use a treadmill, starting slowly increasing the intensity of effort. Remember if you like the exercise program you choose, you will be more likely to stick with it. Another suggestion is to try a "buddy system" to help you get in the habit of exercising. Identify a friend or coworker who also wants to start this good habit, and then urge each other to exercise together.

The time when you're planning to become pregnant is also an excellent time to begin making friends with women who are already pregnant or who have recently had babies. New moms often arrange to walk to the grocery store together with strollers or baby packs or to meet at the playground when the babies become toddlers. You will get to be around adults with at least one similar interest—your babies. You may discover lifelong friendships *and* get some exercise!

KEY THINGS TO REMEMBER
Use safety measures when you exercise:

- Don't overdo it when you're starting out. If it hurts during exercise, stop!
- Make sure your doctor agrees to your starting an exercise program if you haven't been on one.
- It can be dangerous to walk alone in certain places or at night, get your partner or a friend to walk with you.

A Pregnancy Diet

Food. We all need it and we all have opinions about it. You may feel that food is your friend or your enemy. You may feel you think about it too much or not enough. You may think you eat a balanced diet, or feel pretty sure that you have a lousy diet. Your diet may be influenced by personal preference, but you've mainly come to your feelings about food due to your upbringing, perhaps your religious affiliation, and your education. But your education didn't stop after school ended. On a daily basis, you receive new information on food through the media, government reports, commercial advertising, long-term studies, new diet suggestions, new products to try, and scientific breakthroughs . . . The list goes on.

When your goal is healthy eating for pregnancy, how are you to know what's best for you to eat?

Before you're pregnant, you need to be taking in nutritious food to create the best possible environment for your baby. And once you are pregnant, you'll want to know you are supplying the building blocks needed to create a new human being. Naturally, you'll want the best building materials available.

The Best Nutrition

The rules of healthy eating when planning a pregnancy follow the rules for healthy eating for the general public. You're probably familiar with USDA guidelines for healthy eating entitled the "Food Guide Pyramid." It separates foods into four groups. Current literature suggests this pyramid needs to be updated because more and more Americans are relatively inactive and have a high fat intake. However, the four-food-group model is a good place to start understanding what foods to include in your healthy pre-pregnancy diet.

Starting with the group that should be consumed in the largest amount, the food groups are:

- *Grains*, such as pasta, cereal, breads, and rice
- *Fruits and vegetables*
- *Proteins*, from eggs, poultry, meat, fish, nuts, and dry beans
- *Dairy*, in the form of milk, cheeses, and yogurt

Fats, oils, and sweets should also be included, but only in small amounts.

Why are these groups important? Broadly speaking, grains provide your body with vitamin B, minerals, fuel or energy, and fiber. Fruits and vegetables provide fiber, vitamins, and minerals. The dark green leafy vegetables provide important **folic acid**. Protein provides the building materials for new cells, as does dairy. Fats and oils provide fatty acids and vitamins A and E. They are a necessary part of your diet, but only in minuscule amounts. Unfortunately, sweets aren't needed, however much our bodies crave them.

A balanced meal consists of one-third grains, one-third fruits and/or vegetables, one-third protein, and a glass of milk or cup of yogurt. In-between-meal snacks should consist of low-fat grain products such as pretzels or fruits. If you're at your ideal body weight before pregnancy, you should eat three meals a day totaling about 2000 calories. You should also drink six to eight glasses of water each day.

TRY THIS

Write down everything you eat and drink for one complete day. Then assign them to their food groups. Notice where you're missing servings of an important food group.

Grains = 4 or more_____

Fruit/Vegetables = 2 vitamin C fruits/veg.,1 dark green veg, 2 others____

_____

Protein = 2 to 3 servings_____

Dairy = 3 servings (3 8-oz. glasses of milk)_____

Water = 6 to 8 glasses_____

Fats/Oils = sparingly_____

One of the differences in pregnancy versus nonpregnancy diets is that you'll need to increase your intake of foods rich in calcium, iron, and folic acid, three nutrients that are vital to a healthy pregnancy outcome. **It's very important to boost your intake of folic acid *before* you're pregnant.** We'll discuss how to do this in the section on preconceptual counseling. You may also need to increase your intake of fruit, vegetables, and grains to provide your body more fiber, and to reduce your caffeine intake. Eating the right foods will help you be in peak physical condition during your pregnancy and beyond.

However, although you may need to change what you eat when pregnant, you won't be changing how much you eat. Most OB providers will tell you to increase your daily intake of calories by only 300 when you're pregnant.

Special Diets

Many people nowadays experiment with different diets to lose weight or to find one that makes them feel better than others. Some of these diets are regimented and eliminate specific food groups. This is not to say any particular diet is bad for you. The human body can often go without certain nutrients for some time without negative impact. If you follow a diet that avoids carbohydrates, or does not include meat, or dairy, or wheat products—in short, a diet that eliminates or minimizes any of the major food groups—consider finding out what nutrients are not being supplied, and replacing the avoided food with one that is compatible with your diet and supplies the necessary nutrients.

If you're a vegetarian, you are probably already conscientious about getting adequate amounts of nutrition without including meat. You may already take B-12 and calcium supplements. However, you need to consider the body's demand for protein during pregnancy and increase your intake of soybeans or soybean products such as tofu and other high protein sources, such as seeds and nuts. And make sure your health care provider knows about your special preferences in your diet.

Reading Food Labels

There are other ways you can be sure you're eating right for a healthy pregnancy. You can learn how to read the labels now required on all packaged food.

Spend a few minutes studying a food label and it will gradually begin to make more sense to you. Check the serving amount, the number of calories, percentage of fat, amount of protein, and whether it contains any vitamins and minerals. How much you should consume of these items each day is listed near the bottom of each label and is based on an average 2000-calorie diet.

These labels will give you important nutritional information whether you're planning to be pregnant, are already pregnant, breast feeding, or trying to lose weight before or after pregnancy. By using these labels, you'll be able to keep track of your calorie intake. But more important, you can learn how much fat, carbohydrate, and protein is included in your favorite foods. You'll also find out if these favorites contain the vitamins or minerals that are beneficial to your pregnancy. Soon, you'll feel you know which foods to include in your diet and which ones to avoid. Understanding your body's nutritional needs during pregnancy will help you feel confident you're providing everything your baby needs for optimal development and good health.

Before we leave the subject of food, let's not forget your partner. Enlist his support in changing to a diet that includes all the food groups and all the nutrients. Try planning meals together, and consider tasting foods from other lands—after all, you're both on a journey of new experiences.

Reducing Stress in a Stressful World

We have such high expectations for ourselves and for others. We have too little time. Our lives are spent rushing from one commitment to another. And that's just the stress we put on ourselves. Add to that family problems, economic uncertainty, and world events, and stress becomes a heavy burden to try to accommodate.

From a multitude of studies, stress has been linked to illnesses such as high blood pressure, heart attacks, stroke, insomnia, rashes, and muscle pain. Stress can also cause mental illness, such as anxiety attacks, phobias, and depression. Any of these conditions can affect you during your pregnancy. For an easier, more enjoyable pregnancy, the goal should be to alleviate as much stress as possible before the pregnancy begins. How is this possible?

First, try to evaluate how much stress you're under before you get pregnant. You may be completely unaware of the stress in your daily life because you've been handling it for so long. Second, separate out the stress you have control over—such as making too many commitments, or time management—from the stress you have no control over, such as world events or an unexpected illness or loss. Third, see if you can reduce those stress causers that are in your control, and seek help for those stresses out of your control. Learning to manage your stress before you're pregnant will help manage the natural stress that comes with pregnancy and parenthood.

Stress Busters

Here are some suggestions for reducing the stress:

- Exercise, such as walking, is beneficial.
- Increase your amount of rest. Take naps on weekends and go to bed early after a very busy day. Try to get a minimum of eight hours of uninterrupted sleep a night. Some researchers feel Americans, more than people in other countries, suffer from sleep deprivation. Lack of sleep decreases your productivity and, if left unmanaged, can compromise your health.
- Target what's causing your stress. It may stem from a number of things, such as an unsatisfactory career, lack of money, debts, and/or family strife, like a parent's illness or a sibling's dependency. Or it may stem from a partner's previous relationships, an ex-wife, and children. Sometimes just identifying the cause can help reduce the stress.
- Learn to meditate. Explore how busy your mind is and practice turning off the noise caused by a busy world. Get books and articles on other self-help measures that may reduce your stress.
- Journal writing seems to be therapeutic for some people. Putting your thoughts down on paper may decrease your stress and anxiety.
- Do some planning. Stress may be caused by "fear of the unknown." For instance, you may have concerns about how pregnancy and having a baby will impact your finances. It's not too early to start thinking about issues such as working after the baby is born, whether you have the choice of a full- or part-time schedule.

Reducing stress before you begin your pregnancy will make a world of difference in how you feel during this marvelous adventure. Indeed, it may help you have a marvelous adventure. Imagine sailing easily and joyfully through pregnancy and birth rather than creeping along uncertain, beset by worries. Take the steps you need to make your pregnancy as stress-free as possible.

TRY THIS

Ask yourself and your partner the following questions:

What are your work options? Can I return to work after maternity leave? Is my job secure? Does it provide paid maternity leave? Can I work part-time? Flex-time? From home? Can I afford to quit? Do I want a different job or career?

Examine how you feel about working outside the home versus being home with your children. Will one of you stay home or will you use day care? What kind of child care do you prefer? Will it be a private in-home nanny, an au pair, the help of a family member, day care in a home with several other babies, or a licensed day care center? Can your partner adjust his work to take on some or all of the child care?

- You may want to get professional counseling to help you sort out the causes of your stress, especially if you're in a family situation that you feel you cannot manage alone. Ask your doctor for information on hotlines, domestic abuse programs, legal aid services, and counseling.
- Spend time with your friends or family just laughing and relaxing. Take time for yourself, with your partner, and with people whose company you enjoy.
- Ask other couples how they adjusted to the change in their life after a baby.

TRY THIS

In your journal, make a list of the people you feel comfortable with asking for help if you need it. Include their phone numbers so you can quickly and easily reach them. Also list the names of your partner, parents, friends, brothers and sisters, aunts and uncles, teachers, neighbors, coworkers, church, synagogue or mosque acquaintances. You might be surprised at how long the list is.

Your Preconceptual Counseling Appointment

To be certain of all the things you need to take care of before you get pregnant, make an appointment with your OB/GYN provider for a preconceptual office visit. Before you arrive for this visit, you may want to gather information on you and your partner's family health history. Ideally, your partner should also plan to come to the preconceptual visit. You'll both learn a great deal about preparing to conceive your baby and, more important, you'll be starting out together.

TRY THIS

Before the preconceptual visit:

- Prepare information for your doctor or health care provider about your current health in general and past reproductive health.
- Get information about your partner's past medical history and family medical history.
- Ask your parents or family members about your family medical history, immunizations, and childhood diseases.
- List specific conditions you want to investigate and their effect on pregnancy.

At a preconceptual visit, you may have:

1. A physical exam to make sure you're in good health generally and that your reproductive organs appear healthy. This exam will include a pap smear to check that your cervix is healthy.
2. A questionnaire to complete regarding your medical history which inquires about past and current medical problems. You may be asked to give your blood type. The provider will want to know about your environment and health habits, such as diet and amount and type of exercise. He or she may ask you ques-

tions about previous surgeries, your age when you had your first menstrual period, your chosen method of birth control, if you have any chronic illnesses such as diabetes or high blood pressure, and if you have allergies. Your doctor will also want to know if you think you might have problems getting pregnant or if you have ever had a miscarriage.

This medical questionnaire will also ask whether you have had certain childhood illnesses. Ideally, before coming to your preconceptual visit, you should ask your parents which diseases and vaccines you have had. If you need to be vaccinated or have a booster at this preconceptual visit, you may need to wait three months before trying to become pregnant.

The measles, mumps, and rubella (German measles) vaccine is given once and rarely needs a booster. Tetanus and diphtheria shots require a booster every ten years. Hepatitis A, Hepatitis B, influenza, and pneumococcal vaccines may be given if your exposure risk is high, or you are a certain age group that would benefit from this protection. There is a chicken pox vaccine available now, but most women of child-bearing age will have had the disease. You may want to get this vaccine if you cannot find out if you had the disease as a child. Your partner should also try to find out if he's had these diseases or the vaccines, and if not have him discuss with the doctor if he needs to be vaccinated. Chicken pox in adults can be very serious. Having all your vaccines up-to-date will help you feel confident you're ready to proceed to pregnancy.

The medical questionnaire will also ask if you or your partner are around "harmful agents"—such as certain chemicals, heavy metals, lead, and radiation—that can affect your ability to get pregnant or affect the development of the baby. Harmful agents as listed by the National Institute for Occupational Safety and Health (NIOSH) are divided into two categories: male reproductive hazards and female reproductive hazards. See Tables 1–2, 1–3, and 1–4. Male reproductive hazards may affect a man's number or quality of sperm or can affect the sperm's ability to get to the egg to fertilize it. Female reproductive hazards can cause infertility, menstrual cycle changes, miscarriage, premature birth, birth defects, low birth weight, and developmental disorders.

In addition to common hazards found in the workplace, there are also substances used in hobbies or around the home that may be harmful to a pregnancy. For instance, lead is used in smelting metals, paint manufacture, printing, ceramics, and pottery glazing. Think about whether you engage in activities either at work or during leisure time that require the use of harmful agents.

TABLE 1-2. MALE REPRODUCTIVE HAZARDS*				
Observed effects				
Type of Exposure	Lowered number of sperm	Abnormal sperm shape	Altered sperm transfer sexual performance	Altered hormones/
Lead	•	•	•	•
Dibromochloropane	•			
Carbaryl (Sevin)		•		
Toluenediamine and dinitrotoluene	•			
Ethylene dibromide	•	•	•	
Plastic production (styrene and acetone)		•		
Ethlene glycol monoethyl ether	•			
Welding		•	•	
Perchloroethylene			•	
Mercury vapor				•
Heat	•		•	
Military radar	•			
Kepone			•	
Bromine vapor	•	•	•	•
Carbon disulfide				•
2,4-Dichloro-phenoxy acetic acid (2,4-D)		•	•	

*Source: National Institute for Occupational Safety and Health.

TABLE 1-3. CHEMICAL AND PHYSICAL AGENTS THAT ARE REPRODUCTIVE HAZARDS FOR WOMEN IN THE WORKPLACE*

Agent	Observed effects	Potentially exposed workers
Cancer treatment drugs (e.g., methotrexate)	Infertility, miscarriage, birth defects. low birth weight	Health care workers, pharmacists
Certain ethylene glycol ethers such as 2-ethoxyethanol	Miscarriages	Electronic and semiconductor workers
Carbon disulfide (CS_2)	Menstrual cycle changes	Vicose rayon workers
Lead	Infertility, miscarriage, low birth weight, developmental disorders	Battery makers, solderers, welders, radiator repairers, bridge repainters, firing range workers, home remodelers
Ionizing radiation (e.g., X-rays and gamma rays)	Infertility, miscarriage, birth defects. low birth weight, developmental disorders, childhood cancers	Health care workers, dental personnel, atomic workers
Strenuous physical labor (e.g., prolonged standing, heavy lifting)	Miscarriage late in pregnancy, premature delivery	Many types of workers

*Source: National Institute for Occupational Safety and Health.

TABLE 1-4. DISEASE-CAUSING AGENTS THAT ARE REPRODUCTIVE HAZARDS FOR WOMEN IN THE WORKPLACE*

Agent	Observed effects	Potentially exposed workers	Preventive measures
Cytomegalovirus (CMV)	Birth defects, low birth weight, developmental disorders	Health care workers, workers in contact with infants and children	Good hygienic practices such as handwashing
Hepatitis B virus	Low birth weight	Health care workers	Vaccination
Human immuno-deficiency virus (HIV)	Low birth weight, childhood cancer	Health care workers	Practice universal precautions
Human parovirus B-19	Miscarriage	Health care workers, workers in contact with infants and children	Good hygienic practices such as handwashing

TABLE 1-4. (continued)			
Agent	**Observed effects**	**Potentially exposed workers**	**Preventive measures**
Rubella (German measles)	Birth defects, low birth weight	Health care workers, workers in contact with infants and children	Vaccination before pregnancy if no prior immunity
Toxoplasmosis	Miscarriages, birth defects, developmental disorders	Animal care workers, veterinarians	Good hygienic practices such as handwashing
Varicella zoster virus (chicken pox)	Birth defects, low birth weight	Health care workers, workers in contact with infants and children	Vaccination before pregnancy if no prior immunity

*Source: National Institute for Occupational Safety and Health.

Most exposure to harmful agents is taken care of by minimizing contact with the hazardous substance, carefully sealing containers of hazardous agents, wearing protective clothing such as masks and gowns, and by thorough hand washing after contact with harmful agents and before eating and drinking.

Family Medical History

Your preconceptual visit will also include a genetics questionnaire that asks about you and your partner's family medical history. Having this information will help your health care provider assess if there's any chance that your baby may have birth defects or genetic disorders.

If either of you have a family history of a particular disease, you and your partner can be tested for the disorder before conception. There are genetic disorder tests for thalassemia, Tay-Sachs disease, sickle cell disease, hemophilia, muscular dystrophy, cystic fibrosis, Huntington chorea, and Fragile X (a form of mental retardation). Below is a checklist that will help you prepare for the genetics questionnaire. Before trying to answer the questions you may want to ask both sets of parents if they know of family members with any of these diseases.

In reading through this questionnaire, you may find you answered yes to some of the genetic conditions. Keep in mind that this is merely a screening form. Your OB provider can make a better determination of risk after speaking directly with you and your partner. If your OB provider thinks it useful, he or she may refer you to a genetic counselor for advanced preconceptual lab testing and counseling.

TRY THIS

In filling out the genetic self-screening form for births defects and genetic disorders, you may realize you don't know the answers to some of the questions. You may want to ask your parents about them. Completing the checklist before you have a preconceptual visit with your doctor or midwife will help you fill in the gaps for them.

Self-Screening for Risk Factors for Birth Defects and Genetic Disorders

Make a checkmark next to any of these statements that apply to you or your partner.

1. ___I have had a baby with a birth defect.

2. ___I have had more than one miscarriage.

3. ___I have had a stillborn baby.

4. ___I am or will be 35 years old or older when I have the next baby.

5. ___I am from Greek, Italian, Southeast Asian, or Filipino heritage and have a family member with Thalassemia.

6. ___I am from eastern Jewish European (Ashkenazi) or French Canadian descent and have a family member with Tay-Sachs disease.

7. ___I have a blood-related relative with a heart defect that they were born with.

8. ___I have a blood-related relative with Down syndrome.

9. ___I have a blood-related relative with hemophilia or a bleeding disorder.

10. ___I have a blood-related relative with sickle cell disease or sickle cell trait.

11. ___I have a blood-related relative with cystic fibrosis.

12. ___I have a blood-related relative who is mentally retarded.

13. ___I have a blood-related relative who tested positive for fragile X syndrome.

14. ___I have a blood-related relative with spina bifida or a neural tube defect.

15. ___I have a blood-related relative with muscular dystrophy.

16. ___I have a blood-related relative with Huntington disease.

17. ___I have a blood-related relative with some birth defect or inherited disease not mentioned above.

    List the defect or disease _____

18. ___I have been diagnosed with PKU (phenylketonuria).

You and your partner should fill out this form and then take the results to your doctor to review. Let your doctor know the specifics of your medical history.

Checking for Sexually Transmitted Disease

You will be also asked about possible exposure to sexually transmitted diseases (STDs). Many STDs have no symptoms, particularly in women. While no one wants to think they may have a sexually transmitted disease, it's very important to make sure you do not have an STD before you get pregnant. Exposure to any STD may cause health problems for you and your baby. If you feel you've been exposed to an STD either before or while pregnant, tell your doctor or midwife. He or she can easily have you tested and can treat you if necessary. Afterward, you can usually expect a normal pregnancy.

Douching

Talk with your OB Provider about douching. Many women are discouraged from douching just prior to conceiving, during, and after pregnancy. Douching may decrease your body's ability to fight infections like bacterial vaginosis.

Preparation for Pregnancy

After filling out all the forms and answering the questions, your health care provider may provide you with some instructions on how to prepare for your pregnancy.

1. Eliminate poor habits. Your preconceptual health care provider will offer you a weight loss program if you're overweight or may offer you other programs to help you stop smoking or using alcohol or illegal substances, and will offer suggestions for alleviating stress. You will be asked to discontinue any medications that are not approved by your health care provider, including prescription acne medication, medication for psoriasis, or any products containing herbs. Ask about what you can take for headaches and other minor aches and pains. Nonsteroidal anti-inflammatory drugs (NSAID) like Ibuprofen (Advil and Motrin) are under research and are considered something to avoid when planning to conceive or in the first trimester.
2. Eat a healthy diet high in protein, calcium, and iron, and make sure you drink six glasses of water every day. Eating foods high in vitamin C helps with cell development and with absorbing other nutrients. We will talk more about what to eat and drink for a healthy pregnancy later, in Chapter 3.
3. Take folic acid and prenatal vitamins. Your health care provider will prescribe a vitamin specially formulated for pregnancy. The prenatal vitamin includes folic acid. Your health care provider may also want you to take an extra folic acid supplement.
4. Start an exercise program. Most health care professionals in the "baby business" strongly advocate exercise before and during pregnancy. Suggested kinds of exercise are swimming, water aerobics, yoga, and walking.

Folic acid is a synthetic B vitamin also called *folate* in its natural form. **It is important to have an adequate amount of folic acid in your body before you conceive** because it's needed soon after conception to form the neural tubes of your developing baby. When these tubes don't form properly, there are "neural tube defects," more commonly known as spina bifida, or anencephaly. Realizing the importance of folic acid in women's diets, in 1992 the FDA began requiring that folic acid be added to products such as breads, cereals, and other grain products. Folic acid or folate is also found naturally in leafy vegetables, beans (legumes), citrus fruits, and whole grains.

5. Think about preferences in your prenatal care and baby's delivery. You might not think that you have preferences or be aware that you have options. In fact you have several choices in professional prenatal, delivery, and postpartum care. Your health care provider may ask you to start thinking about the kind of delivery you'd like to have.

Creating Your Birth Plan

To help you sort out what you would prefer for your baby's delivery, we suggest as one tool a "birth plan"—a plan of birth preparation that has become popular in the last few years. The idea is to *plan* how you would like your pregnancy and childbirth to go. In a birth plan's barest sense, this means knowing where, with whom, and how you would like to go through labor and delivery—the birth of your baby.

On most journeys, you want to get from point A to point B. On a pregnancy journey, you will first need to decide what you want point B to be. Point B is where you want to have the baby and how. Point A is what health care professional can provide that type of delivery. Knowing where you want to deliver may seem like putting the cart before the horse, especially when you aren't even pregnant yet. However, the "where and with whom" of your birth options may be constrained by the kind of insurance you carry, the hospitals or birthing centers located in your area, the availability of medical choices from your OB provider, and by your health status.

During your preconceptual visit you should find out your insurance options for prenatal care and delivery. Ideally, you want a health insurance policy that offers a preconceptual visit, genetic testing, prenatal care, ultrasound, infertility diagnosis and treatment, postpartum care, and a choice of:

- Doctor or midwife
- Hospital, birthing center, or home delivery
- Birthing room or a standard delivery room
- Medication-free birth or use of pain medications

Your birth plan can be as brief as deciding where to have the baby and with whom. Or it can be as detailed as choosing everything you would like to happen during your pregnancy and delivery. You may feel that for now you have no idea how to make these decisions about what you prefer. We'll explain all of these preferences. We call them "preferences" because they are what you would prefer given a complication-free pregnancy, labor, and delivery. Keep in mind that doctors and midwives reserve the right to override the wishes of the couple if you or your baby's health is at risk.

Let's talk about the different types of health care professionals who deliver babies. This will help you understand your options.

Planning Your Delivery

Care by an Obstetrician

Licensed medical physicians who provide prenatal care and deliver babies are usually obstetricians. They specialize in the care of women during pregnancy and are board certified in prenatal care, delivery, and care of gynecological (women's) issues. Obstetricians, or OB/GYNs, provide prenatal care, with or without the assistance of a nurse practitioner, in a professional office. Many are trained as surgeons to perform cesarean deliveries and obstetric and gynecological procedures.

An OB/GYN nurse practitioner is a registered nurse with specialized training in pregnancy and is fully versed in prenatal obstetrical care. Many NPs have master's degrees in obstetrics and women's health. A nurse practitioner can provide prenatal care, diagnose problems with pregnancy, and prescribe medications. Many nurse practitioners focus on educating you and your partner about pregnancy and work closely with an obstetrician.

In 2001, the CDC reports that 91.3 percent of all births in the United States occurred with the assistance of a doctor in a hospital setting.[1]

Most hospitals now have birthing suites—rooms designed to look like a birthing center room or even a hotel room. The more medical-looking equipment is hidden from view but available when needed. In general, you're encouraged to remain upright and let gravity help the birth progress, especially in early labor. You can walk around the room and hallway, sit in a chair, and take showers to make going through the labor more comfortable. It's likely you'll be given fluids intravenously, which may limit your movement somewhat but keep you from getting dehydrated. It's very important to be adequately hydrated to maintain your strength for the physical work of labor.

When the need arises, this bedroomlike setting can quickly be transformed into a hospital room equipped to handle most birth situations. Your partner or other family members can stay with you through the labor and delivery, unless there's an emergency situation.

Having a doctor-assisted hospital birth means having the option to use an *epidural* or pain-blocking medications during your labor. An epidural is a medication delivered to the lower back. It can help you tolerate labor pain and is available should the labor become too difficult. Many women feel strongly about the benefits of an epidural; others do not. (See Chapter 7, "Pain Relief Options.")

Many couples feel the biggest advantage of a doctor-assisted hospital birth is the fact that if any part of your labor goes awry and emergency intervention or a cesarean becomes necessary, the most up-to-date medical technology and personnel are right there to take care of the problem.

In a hospital delivery, you and the baby will usually stay two days after a vaginal birth and three to four days after a cesarean birth, providing there are no complications. The hospital staff will continually check you and your baby for problems and ensure that you are both doing well after the delivery.

Finding a Doctor

Most insurance plans allow you to choose your doctor, but you may have to choose from a list of specifically contracted doctors called "participating" or "par" doctors. Currently, most private OB/GYNs belong to group practices that are contracted by HMOs. Many doctors are in such large group practices that you may not get to know them all. You may opt to see different OB/GYNs for each prenatal visit to get a feel for the one you're most comfortable with and then request that doctor for future visits. However, even a doctor. in a solo practice occasionally has another physician covering for him or her in a variety of situations. The doctor you hoped would do your delivery is not always going to be available when you go into labor. For both private practice and HMO obstetrics providers, in most cases, whoever is on call at the time of your labor and delivery will be your doctor at the time of delivery.

Care by a Midwife

Certified Nurse Midwives. Certified Nurse Midwives (CNMs) have a Master of Science degree in nurse midwifery and women's health care and are certified by the American College of Nurse-Midwives. In addition to delivery, most CNMs are trained in immediate neonatal care and breast-feeding technique. They give the baby its initial examination after delivery and provide coaching for successful breast-feeding.

There are licensed CNMs in every state. Some midwifery practices deliver only in hospitals, some have separate birthing centers, and some will deliver in your home. You can look for them in your local yellow pages or go to the ACNM Web site (American College of Nurse-Midwives) on the Internet. There are ACNM chapters in every state.

Delivery of a baby at a birthing center with a CNM is usually less expensive than a hospital delivery. Many HMOs and other insurance plans will cover the cost of birthing centers and midwives, thus allowing you to choose this kind of delivery. If you wish to have a home birth with a midwife, you should check your insurance policy to see if the cost of home birth is reimbursable. If it is not and you still want a home birth, you can choose to pay for the home birth yourself, but you can still use your insurance to cover the cost of hospitalization if that becomes necessary.

Lay Midwives. Lay midwives are midwives without formal medical training and usually "on-the-job" training. They have learned by apprenticing to other midwives or are self-taught. These midwives do not have a nursing degree in midwifery. They are not constrained by protocols or the health care system. Most are found through word of mouth. The material in this book refers only to certified nurse midwives.

If you were to choose a midwife for your baby's delivery, your prenatal care can take place at the birthing center or in the offices of the midwife's practice. You may deliver your baby in the birthing center, a hospital, or in your home.

The practice of midwifery is based on the belief that women are designed to have babies and that birth is a "normal" event. Nearly 10 percent of births in the United States are midwife-delivered, and this number is growing.[2] Women are choosing midwives for a variety of reasons, but one of the primary ones is a desire to have a natural birth and to avoid the use of pain medication.

Midwives believe nonmedicating pain alleviating techniques such as change of position, water therapy, massage, and the upright position enable women to deliver their babies "naturally." Some women feel midwives take more time with their patients and are better able to encourage the active participation of the mother in labor. Many women choose a midwife for their deliveries because they feel the extra time midwives take allow them to listen to their concerns and this helps minimize the fear of giving birth and thus shortens labor.

Epidurals are not available in birthing centers, but if you were to find labor unbearably painful, you can ask to be transferred to the hospital. Some midwives offer analgesics to help with the pain if you want to continue labor at the birthing center. They will usually encourage you to walk, move, or change position frequently and to use the shower or whirlpool to alleviate the pain of labor and move the labor along more quickly toward delivery. You are free to eat, but most women are not hungry during labor. You are asked to drink water to remain hydrated, and will receive an IV if you cannot keep liquids down.

Another medication not available in birthing centers is oxytocin (Pitocin). Oxytocin induces labor contractions, trying to "jump start" a labor that has stalled. If your labor fails to progress, you can be transferred to a hospital where your midwife or in many cases her backup obstetrician can give you oxytocin and continue managing your delivery. (See Chapter 7— Failure to Progress)

Midwives only deliver mothers by vaginal birth. If you were to develop complications of labor and/or need a cesarean section, your midwife will transfer the delivery to a physician. Midwives are very comfortable in detecting deviations from normal birth in plenty of time to safely transfer your care to a physician. They can manage the minor complications of labor.

Delivery by a midwife at a freestanding birthing center is only for women who have minor or no preexisting medical conditions. But you can probably choose to have a midwife delivery with the following complications: Rh negative, over 35 years of age with a first baby, or if you have a history of miscarriages. If you have a medical condition not related to pregnancy, you can often deliver with a midwife if the condition is stabilized. For instance, a midwife can deliver you if you have diabetes that is controlled with diet and the baby appears to have no complications. However, some of these conditions require that a midwife delivery take place in the hospital, by a midwife with immediate physician backup.

After delivery in a birthing center, you may remain at the center for up to 12 hours, but you'll need to stay a minimum of four hours. This is to ensure that you and the baby have recovered from the birth, that you're able to shower and eat, and that you can nurse with confidence.

Some medical practices offer care with both a physician and a licensed midwife. Either one can deliver your baby. Often, the deliveries are performed in a hospital setting with the "natural" childbirth philosophy, and many of the patient's choices are accommodated (see Table 1-5).

TABLE 1-5. DIFFERENCES AND SIMILARITIES BETWEEN PHYSICIAN AND CERTIFIED MIDWIFE DELIVERY

Physician Delivery	Midwife Delivery
1. Prenatal care in doctor's office.	1. Prenatal care in midwife's office, birthing center
2. Delivery in hospital	2. Delivery in hospital, birthing center or home
3. Birthing room	3. Birthing room
4. Encourage movement during labor	4. Encourage movement during labor
5. No food or drink, IV if needed	5. Food and drink, IV if needed
6. Epidurals or analgesics for pain	6. No epidurals, but analgesics for pain
7. Can handle any kind of delivery	7. Can only deliver vaginally
8. Two to three days postpartum in hospital	8. Four to 12 hours postpartum in birthing center

Home Delivery with a Midwife

You may want to have your baby at home. You may feel that you will be more comfortable in your own environment, be less inhibited during labor and delivery, or be more in control of the birth event if it occurs at home. Like birthing center deliveries, home births are only available to women without pregnancy complications. Also, home births are not always covered by major medical insurance plans. You'll need to review your coverage.

With a home birth, your prenatal visits will usually take place in the midwifery group's office or birthing center. The midwife or her assistant will make at least one visit to your home before the birth to make sure the environment is safe and conducive for a home delivery and that you've assembled the necessary supplies, most of which are typically in the home already. The midwife provides medical supplies.

When labor begins, your midwife and an assistant will come to your home. They will have already instructed you on how to prepare your bedroom and bed and what supplies to have on hand for the baby. Home midwives use the same nonmedicating, pain-alleviating techniques as midwives in a birthing center. As in birthing centers, they're prepared to have you transported to the nearest hospital if they feel it's warranted. After the birth, the nurse midwife and assistant will stay with you for several hours or until they're sure you and the baby are fine. There must be an adult staying with you for up to 72 hours after the birth, or the midwife will arrange to have you transported to a hospital. The midwife will recommend you take the baby to a pediatrician the next day. They will return to your home about a week later for a postpartum checkup.

Doula, a Mother's Helper

Doula is a Greek word meaning "mothering the mother." Doulas are usually nonprofessionals who have been trained to help you in a specific situation, usually in labor. However, there are two types of doulas. A *birth doula* can help you during labor and delivery. A *postpartum doula* helps you during the postpartum period. Some doulas function as both birth and postpartum doulas.

Birth doulas are familiar with the birthing process. Despite birth preparation classes, first-time parents-to-be are often nervous about what their particular labor will look and feel like, and doulas can be a great comfort to you and your partner, who may feel helpless in the face of your obvious pain. These women can help when your partner doesn't feel confident about coaching the delivery. Some doulas are also massage therapists who can provide a measure of physical relief to you during labor.

Birth doulas:

- Meet you both before the due date
- Provide comfort measures during your labor and birth
- Help you with breast-feeding immediately after birth
- Follow up with a postpartum visit one week after the delivery
- Are available by phone for any questions or concerns

Often, birth doulas hold a first meeting on the phone and then two or more meetings in person to give you time to discuss your birth plan and see if you're comfortable working with each other. When you're in early labor, your doula may meet you at the hospital or come to your home and accompany you to the hospital. She will remain with you throughout labor and delivery.

Hospital studies have found that having birth doulas present at births reduces the number of cesarean sections, epidurals, and the need for oxytocin by about 50 percent. On average, the duration of labor is shortened by 25 percent, or about two hours.[3]

Some hospitals and OB/GYN practices encourage women to consider the support provided by a birth doula for their deliveries, and even provide doula training. Check with the hospital you plan to deliver at. There may be some restrictions about a doula's role during delivery.

Postpartum doulas act as mother's helpers after the parents and baby come home from the hospital or birthing center. They can help with breast-feeding counseling, cooking, cleaning, baby care, night-time feeding shifts, or first-time parent nervousness. Postpartum doulas are especially helpful when the mother has limited family support in the area.

If having a doula appeals to you, ask your health care provider for information and a referral or check on the National Doula Web site. Doulas can also be found by word of mouth. Some insurance plans may cover doula service, and some hospitals offer these services as part of the hospital fee.

You now have the information to begin to see where your preferences lie. Do not hesitate to gather more information from your health care professionals, the testimony of friends and family, and even from other sources at the library or on the Internet. The most important thing to realize is that you have options about how your pregnancy and delivery will go. You can choose what sounds right for you. When you know you have a say in how your care will go, you will feel empowered. You should have the birth you want to have.

Childbirth Preparation Techniques

While you're making your birth plan, we suggest you look into the philosophies of several childbirth preparation techniques. To be effective, all of these techniques require you to start practicing their methods before the third trimester.

Three of these techniques are ASPO/Lamaze, the Bradley method, and HypnoBirthing. All of them teach you how to be an active participant in your labor, how your body works during labor, and recommend exercises that may decrease the pain and shorten labor. The goal for each of these methods is that you have a personal, natural, and joyful birth experience. We recommend that you explore these techniques to see if you feel they fit your hopes for your birth experience and will make your birth journey easier.

TRY THIS

Make a birth plan by writing down the following preferences, realizing that they are your preferences and if complications occur your baby and your health are the major concern:

- Place of delivery: hospital, birthing center, or home birth
- Professional for prenatal care and delivery: doctor or midwife
- Labor Doula: yes or no
- Childbirth preparation method: ASPO/Lamaze, Bradley, Hypno-Birthing, other
- Prefer pain medication: yes or no
- Prefer vaginal birth after a cesarean section: yes or no
- Prefer not to have an episiotomy: yes or no
- Planning to breast-feed: yes or no
- Do you want your male baby circumcised: yes or no

Note: You may not feel ready to decide on all of these factors. And, as you go through your pregnancy, you may change your mind about your initial preferences. You should always feel you have the right to do so.

Health Insurance Coverage

Now that you have some idea of your birth choices, you'll need to make sure your insurance will cover your preferences for prenatal care, type of provider, and place of delivery. If your current insurance doesn't allow for your choice and you're still committed to a certain kind of birth, you will either have to try to find another insurance plan that provides the coverage you want before you get pregnant or budget to cover the cost yourself. Some health plans have very strict preexisting conditions clauses, and pregnancy may be considered a preexisting condition, meaning the coverage will be limited or that your pregnancy will not be covered.

Knowing what you can expect from your plan will help you with critical decision making. You and your partner should get answers to the following questions about your insurance *before becoming pregnant.*

Insurance Question Checklist

1. Do you have health insurance that covers pregnancy, prenatal care, and delivery?
2. Is it group insurance through your employer or your partner's employer?
3. Do you cover each other on your health insurance?
4. Are you covered as "a significant other" or "domestic partner"? (You should be aware that many insurance companies do not allow coverage for these situations.)
5. If you don't have group insurance, can you get a single policy?
6. Is pregnancy a preexisting condition and thus not covered by your insurance if you are pregnant before you get coverage?
7. Is it comprehensive, meaning does it cover everything? If not what isn't covered?
8. Does it have a deductible? What will be your financial contribution?
9. Does it have a dollar limit of coverage per year?
10. Does it allow you the choice to deliver in a hospital, birthing center, or home birth?
11. Does it allow you to choose your OB/GYN?
12. Does it cover infertility diagnosis and treatment?
13. Does it cover the cost of a birth and/or postpartum doula?

Medicaid

We strongly recommend you get health insurance before becoming pregnant if you can afford it. If you're unable to afford any type of insurance, find out if you're eligible for Medicaid, which is government-funded health care. You can contact your local health department listed in the phone book. Many women do not realize that Medicaid is available even to some women who work.

Disability Insurance

You may want to check if your employer offers disability insurance before getting pregnant. If not, you may want to buy a separate plan. Disability insurance can help you financially if you have a complication and are unable to work during your pregnancy or if you have a major medical complication after delivery and cannot return to work. If problems arise in your pregnancy, your doctor may prescribe long-term bed rest, meaning you will not be able to work. Disability insurance will protect you from a complete loss of income. Talk with your benefit administrator at work or call the health plan directly.

Enjoy Your Pre-Pregnancy Period

You're planning to embark on a brand new life—being pregnant. This new life will have many of its own rewards, but it's worthwhile to acknowledge the changes brought with this new phase of life.

One of the most important things you can do for yourself and your partner before pregnancy is to savor the things you enjoy now. Many of the following events may become more difficult during your pregnancy and after the arrival of your baby.

- Consider taking a relaxing vacation before you try to get pregnant. You may find a vacation a bit more challenging during your pregnancy and for quite a while after the baby has come. Pregnancy can bring discomforts such as nausea, interrupted sleep, and stress, which can make a vacation less restful. Of course, you won't have to give up vacations for the next 20 years, but once you're pregnant, and certainly once you have children, you may find that vacations are not as carefree as they once were.
- Engage in the activities you enjoy, such as going to concerts or movies. It may not be as comfortable to do them when you have to get up frequently to use the bathroom. And once the baby arrives, it may be hard to find reliable babysitters. The serious

patron of the arts will find ways to get to theatrical events during pregnancy and after giving birth, but for many the effort will outweigh the payoff, and going out to the movies or theater is likely to decrease, at least for a while.

- Get as much sleep as you can. Indulge in Sunday afternoon naps; go to bed early and sleep late whenever you can. Once you're pregnant, you may find you don't sleep through the night anymore, your body will ache in new places, and you won't be able to sleep on your stomach, if you prefer that position. Perhaps worst is that you might need to get up to urinate several times in the night. And after the baby arrives, there will be a period when you have to get up regularly at night to tend to him or her. All these changes will alter your sleeping habits for a long time.

- Eat delicious and nutritious dinners, either prepared by you or your partner, if you both enjoy cooking, or at restaurants. During pregnancy, food you once loved may seem distasteful. What's more, the nausea you experience in the first few months of pregnancy may make eating out nearly unbearable. And, as the fetus grows, the room in your stomach may seem to decrease. Finally, once your baby arrives the chance to sit through a meal without jumping up to check on a fussy infant, fetch milk for a toddler, mop up a spill, or tend to a child asking for help in the bathroom may make you look back wistfully at premotherhood days.

Communicating with Each Other

We end this chapter with some things for you and your partner to think about as you get ready to start on this journey together. There are going to be fears of the unknown. We list some of these fears because we want you to know it is not uncommon to have these feelings. Recognize them as fears of the unknown, then share your concerns with your partner. These fears are just that, fears. Remind yourself that they are either not real or probably overexaggerated.

Common fears expectant couples have include:

- Body changes—that at times may make you feel you're unrecognizable

- Becoming unattractive to your partner
- Changing relationships in a negative way
- Changing lifestyles that you cannot handle
- Changing environments that you are not comfortable with
- The huge responsibility of caring for a helpless human being
- Negotiating time off from work will make work seem less important
- Not having enough money
- The pain of childbirth
- The possibility of a miscarriage, still birth, baby with a problem
- Not being a good parent

You Can Do This!

Planning to have a baby can be fun, but it can also be overwhelming. Don't let the planning for your pregnancy take over your entire life. Other areas of your life need attention too, like caring for your partner. You need to keep checking with each other to make sure the journey is going in a way that you both want it to go. This is something you want to do, something you should enjoy.

We don't have to convince you of the joys of parenthood. If you're reading this book, we assume you've already done some thinking about it. If you've cared for friends' or siblings' babies, you already have an inkling of the joy caring for your own baby will bring. From merely holding a sleeping baby in your arms to that first day when your baby smiles at you in recognition, and later when your baby reaches for you, there are millions of occasions for happiness with your child.

As mothers of school-age children and teenagers, we can assure you that raising children gets better and better. As a child grows, many parents remark upon the wonder they feel at being loved by a baby and then by the child. They marvel at the realization that they brought this new being into the world, someone who didn't exist before. Share your dreams about future joys as well as fears with your partner, and give him the opportunity to express his feelings too.

We wish you *bon voyage!*

2

The Start of Your Journey: Trying to Get Pregnant

 Sonia's Journal

Dear Journal,

I'm still in shock that I'm finally pregnant. I want this journal to help me remember that it wasn't easy to get to this place I thought most couples just stop their birth control and boom, they're pregnant. That's the way it was for Linda and Rick. They hadn't even planned on being pregnant so soon after they got married. Linda said it happened when she was switching from the pill to a diaphragm. But they are excited about being parents. That sure wasn't our experience. Brian and I tried for about nine months and then Dr. Joseph recommended we go to Dr. Baker, an infertility specialist. She had me do several tests, told me I had problems with a hormone imbalance, and put me on medication. It was a very intense time, with many trips to the doctor, and it wasn't completely covered by our insurance. But we knew it would be worth it. And it worked! We're going to have a baby!

You've done a lot of preparation for your journey. You obtained the health insurance coverage you need and had a preconceptual visit with an OB/GYN Provider. You're exercising and eating healthier foods. If you smoke, you have limited the amount of smoking or cut it out entirely. You are taking a multivitamin with folic acid and have cut back your consumption of alcohol and caffeine. You're ready to try to get pregnant. Now, it's time to stop using your method of birth control.

You can stop most types of contraception on your own, but some birth control methods require a "waiting period" before you can try to get pregnant. The reason is, your body needs time to return to its normal balance without the influence of contraceptive hormones. During this waiting period, you'll need to use a barrier form of birth control, such as a diaphragm or condom. To remove other forms of contraception—such as IUDs and Norplant—you'll need assistance from your OB provider at his or her office. Your OB provider should be able to give you an estimate of how long it will take to get pregnant after stopping birth control and how soon to schedule a revisit if you do not get pregnant.

Barrier and Hormone-Based Contraceptives

Diaphragms, cervical caps, sponges, or condoms—the so-called "barrier contraceptives"—don't require a waiting period. Simply stop using them if your health care provider agrees that you are otherwise ready for pregnancy.

In contrast, your OB provider may ask you to use condoms or another barrier type of contraception after you've stopped using hormone-based contraceptives, since the latter alter the level of hormones that would normally be produced by your body. You might have to undergo this suggested regimen until you have at least three normal menstrual cycles. For many women this is usually about five to six months. You may experience some spotting or unexpected bleeding or missed periods for a couple of months before your menstrual cycles return to normal.

The hormone-based contraceptives include:

- Birth control pills
- Contraceptive patch

- Depo provera injections (your doctor will stop giving you injections)
- Norplant (you'll need to have it removed during a doctor's office visit)

Intrauterine Devices

You'll need to schedule an appointment to remove your IUD. Ideally, this is done during your menstrual period, when your cervix, the opening to your uterus, is more relaxed and open. Your OB provider will want to check you for minor infections and may want you to use barrier protection for contraception for three months after removal of the IUD. This will allow your body to return to normal function. After your IUD is removed, you may notice slightly more bleeding with the first period.

Taking the Mystery Out of Conception: How Pregnancy Occurs

During intercourse, millions of sperm are released from the penis and enter the vagina, optimally near the cervix, which is the opening to the uterus (see Figure 2-1). Once through the cervix, the sperm must travel up into the two fallopian tubes, one of which contains an egg that has been released from one of the ovaries that month. Only one sperm is able to fully penetrate the egg and fertilize it. The fertilized egg becomes an embryo within a few days. About seven days after fertilization, the embryo descends into the uterus and is implanted in the lining of the uterus.

Changes in the level of certain hormones control each of these steps. If any part of this sequence does not occur, a pregnancy in the uterus will not occur. With all that is involved, it's amazing that anyone does manage to get pregnant. Statistically, healthy women in their early 20s have a 20 to 35 percent chance of conceiving each month they try.[1] While those odds seem low, most couples successfully become pregnant within six months of trying to conceive.

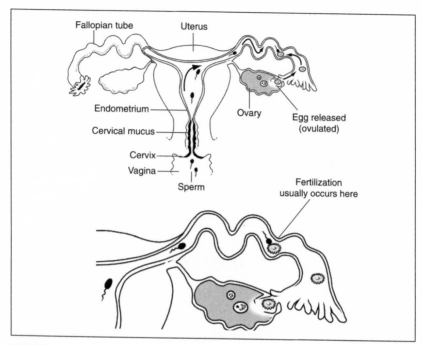

FIGURE 2-1   (Top) The female reproductive tract. (Bottom) The point where fertilization usually occurs.

Hormones and Pregnancy

In this selection we want you to understand the importance of hormones and their effects on your body because it will help you understand what your doctor is referring to during your medical treatment. Hormones control the female reproductive system. The key reproductive hormones are listed here:

- *Estrogen* and its partner *progesterone* signal the uterine lining to thicken and mature in preparation for a fertilized egg. Progesterone also signals the uterus to shed its lining during menstruation and to start the new menstrual cycle.
- *Follicular-stimulating hormone* (FSH), which signals the ovaries to prepare to mature an egg prior to ovulation.
- *Luteinizing hormone* (LH), which triggers the release of the mature egg into the fallopian tube.

- *Gonadotropin-releasing hormone* (GnRH) helps the pituitary gland produce more FSH and LH.
- *Human chorionic gonadotropin* (hCG) is made by the fertilized egg. It signals your ovaries to produce more estrogen and progesterone to maintain the pregnancy.

When there are any alterations in the balance of these hormones, problems with fertility may occur.

Ovulation and the Menstrual Cycle

Pregnancy can only occur when you have ovulated (or released an egg) from one of your ovaries and the egg is fertilized. Every month, under the influence of FSH, your ovaries select an egg that will mature and ovulate. Your ovaries begin maturing an egg and increase the estrogen levels. Changing levels of estrogen and progesterone cause the lining of the uterus to thicken in preparation for implantation and receiving the embryo. This lining, or *endometrium*, contains nutrients that will sustain a fertilized egg once it implants there.

A surge of LH triggers ovulation and the egg is released from the ovary into the tube. You may be aware of the egg leaving the ovary when you feel minor changes, such as very light cramps, or twinges in the abdomen. This is called Mittelschmerz or midcycle pain. You may also notice an increase in clear, slippery cervical mucus that enhances sperm travel through the uterus.

When the egg is released, it enters the nearby fallopian tube where sperm fertilizes it and conception occurs. If the egg is not fertilized within 12 to 24 hours it is reabsorbed by the body. When the egg is no longer in the uterus or fallopian tubes and you're having your period, pregnancy usually will not occur.

When an egg is fertilized it usually moves within a week into the uterus and implants into the endometrium of the uterus. You might believe you're menstruating when in fact you are experiencing spotting, which typically occurs when an embryo has implanted in the uterus. If your period is late or you're spotting you may be pregnant. With a blood test, your OB provider can confirm your pregnancy.

Your Cycle

The key to determining when you're most likely to conceive, and when you are not, is knowing what a normal menstrual cycle is for you. Determining this may take a few months if you were using birth control that altered your normal cycle. It's one reason your OB provider may ask you to use alternate, non-hormone-based contraceptives for a few months before you try to become pregnant.

A woman's cycle generally is every 28 days, although you can have a cycle that is as short as 21 days and as long as 35 days. Let's review the 28 day cycle. It transpires as follows:

- The first day of the cycle, day one, your period begins.
- About five to seven days later the menstrual period stops. The uterine lining has already begun to thicken in preparation for the arrival of another fertilized egg. At the same time, the follicles of the other ovary begin to mature another egg. The ovaries generally alternate monthly in releasing the eggs.
- About 13 or 14 days from the *start* of the menstrual period, the egg is mature enough to be released from the ovary into the fallopian tube. This is *ovulation*.
- Ideally, ovulation occurs between the 13th and 15th day. Because the time of ovulation may vary from month to month, the fertile period is usually calculated from day 10, from the start of the period, to day 17.
- Coitus, or sexual intercourse, must take place during this fertile period if conception is to occur. Sperm can survive approximately three days in a woman's body, but the egg can survive only 12 to 24 hours.

As you can see, predicting the exact time when a couple should have sex is very difficult. Pregnancy occurs most often when regular, repeated coitus begins *before* ovulation. To confirm what your cycle range is and the best time to get pregnant talk with your OB provider.

Catching the Egg: Determining Ovulation

You may want to chart your cycle to learn when you ovulate. With this information, you can begin having coitus or intercourse several days before you expect the next ovulation.

There are several "self-assessments" you can do to chart your menstrual cycle. These will be especially important if you discover you aren't getting pregnant after having stopped your form of contraception, usually more than six months. The information gathered in the self-assessments will help your OB provider evaluate why you may be having difficulty conceiving. Even if you don't expect any trouble becoming pregnant, by studying your cycle you can learn the best time to have intercourse with your partner and achieve a pregnancy.

Fertility Calendar. One self-assessment is a fertility calendar. Each month, mark down on a calendar the following:

- The first day of your menstrual period.
- The day it ends.
- Start estimating when your next period will start. For instance, if your periods are usually 28 to 30 days apart, count off 28 to 30 days and make a mark which indicates your prediction.
- Count back 14 days to estimate when you will ovulate.

Let's say the first day of your period in the month of May was May 1, and your period lasted until May 5. If your period takes place every 28 to 30 days, your next period should start between May 29 and May 31. That means you will probably ovulate on May 14, give or take a few days on either side.

Cervical Mucus Assessment. Another self-assessment is to note, on the same calendar, changes in your cervical mucus. Your body secretes more cervical mucus just prior to ovulation. And not only is there more mucus—it's thicker and slippery. This thicker, slippery, sticky mucus makes it easier for the sperm to swim through the cervix on its way through the uterus to the fallopian tubes. To do this assessment, you cannot be squeamish about touching your body:

- Use a tissue to wipe your vaginal area prior to urinating. You will see a clear or sometimes light yellow discharge, which is mucus. Hold it between your thumb and finger and try to see how sticky and stretchy it is.
- Start by checking your mucus on approximately day 12 of your cycle (the 12th day from the start of your last period).

- Write on your calendar when you started checking and when it's thickest and sticky.
- **Tip:** Don't check your mucus after sex.

Body Temperature Assessment. An additional self-assessment is to check your basal body temperature every day at the same time. When you ovulate, your body temperature goes up about 0.5 of a degree

Keep a thermometer next to your bed. Also keep paper and pencil and/or graph paper if you want to plot the temperature changes (one axis for temperature and the other for the date).

- Take your temperature by mouth every morning (ideally at the same time each morning, with the same thermometer) before getting out of bed or having anything to eat or drink. Record it.
- Do this every day for one to two months. You should see a fairly steady temperature throughout the month, except for a drop just prior to starting your menstrual period and a rise just after you ovulate.

You can use all three self-assessments to see if they predict your ovulation about the same time. Share this information with your health care provider at your next office visit.

You can buy an Ovulation Predictor Kit at the drugstore. This is a home urine test to detect for the luteinizing hormone, which causes the release of a mature egg from the ovary. Follow the detailed instructions to see when you're ovulating. Some recommend that it is best to use this test between 2 p.m. and 7 p.m.

Once you can gauge when you're ovulating, you can start planning to have more frequent sex during these fertile periods.

Frequency of Sex and the Best Position for Conception

In your quest for a baby, remember that sex is referred to as making love. You don't want to forget to seek that special connection with your partner, especially when creating a new life together.

You may be concerned that having sex too often will deplete your partner's supply of sperm. Although males make new sperm continually, daily sex can reduce sperm levels. However, having sex every other day or more than once a week during the fertile period seems to have some beneficial effect on sperm mobility, or how well the sperm wriggle about and move forward. In fact, sperm mobility has been found to be one of the most important factors for successful fertilization. It is usually more important than how many sperm the male ejaculates.

Some believe the best position for conception is the "missionary" position, with you on your back below your partner and facing him. This allows gravity to help bring sperm through the cervix and closer to the fallopian tubes. In some cases you may increase your chances of becoming pregnant by remaining flat on your back for 20 to 30 minutes after sex, to allow the semen to remain near the cervix.

KEY THINGS TO REMEMBER

- Do not use lubricating solutions; they trap the sperm and may even kill them.
- If you must use a lubricant, use a small amount of vegetable or olive oil. A water-soluble lubricant like K-Y jelly can kill the sperm. Petroleum jelly or Vaseline is not a good choice.
- Do not douche. Douching washes the sperm away from the cervix and can change the normal pH (acid or alkaline) of your vagina. Douching can also destroy sperm.
- Do not use a tampon to keep semen in the vagina. The tampon will absorb the semen and keep it away from the cervix.

Keep in mind that trying to get pregnant should be fun. You can now make love without worrying about birth control! You probably won't have that opportunity too many times in your life.

You may want to have a couple of home pregnancy tests on hand. When purchasing them, check the expiration date on the container. Follow the directions closely. Home tests are very reliable if used as directed. Taking a home pregnancy test allows you to be the first to know you're pregnant!

If You Don't Have a Male Partner

If you want to have a baby but don't have a male partner who can provide the sperm for fertilization, you can talk with your OB or infertility provider about artificial insemination with donor sperm from a reputable sperm bank. Sperm is easily purchased, but you may want to talk with your OB or infertility provider about a sperm bank that closely monitors and screens male donors.

Donor sperm is sometimes used to help couples have a baby when the male partner has a low sperm count or no sperm. However, it's also available when there is no male partner involved. Be sure to check your insurance for coverage of infertility, including artificial insemination with donor sperm and for any regulations on waiting periods for infertility services.

When Getting Pregnant Isn't Easy

Perhaps you've been trying to get pregnant for six to eight months without results. You may have, or you're beginning to have, some concerns about being able to get pregnant. Or perhaps you already know that getting pregnant may be difficult for you, or you've been pregnant before and have lost the baby in a miscarriage.

The second half of this chapter we'll go into and explain the various problems some couples have when trying to get pregnant. It will help you and your partner understand how you can work with your OB provider or infertility specialist to solve your infertility problem. The steps toward becoming pregnant may include the expertise of specialists dedicated to helping couples overcome more complicated problems with infertility. Their mission is to help the two of you get pregnant and have a baby.

According to the Center for Disease Control, infertility affected about 6.1 million women in the United States in 1995, or about 10 to 15 percent of the population.[2] Half of these couples will go on to conceive a baby.[3] Because of rapid advances in fertility treatments, the number of couples unable to conceive will steadily shrink in the coming years.

What You Both Can Do to Improve Fertility

To help you get pregnant, it's important that you avoid tobacco, drugs, and alcohol. These chemicals adversely affect conception by reducing sperm and egg *quality*. Both sperm and eggs are delicate cells. They may develop abnormally because of exposure to toxic substances.

If you smoke, take drugs, or are taking medications or supplements you haven't told your OB or infertility provider about, you may have problems becoming pregnant. Stopping these harmful activities may be all you need to do to get your pregnancy started. By avoiding these toxins to your system, you'll be improving your health and giving your baby a better start.

What Your Partner Can Do

Reduce (Sperm) Scrotal Temperature. Sperm is produced in the sacs called *testes*, which are outside the male body because they do not survive in normal core body temperature. Sperm quality and count may be affected by holding the scrotum (which holds the testis) up against the warmer parts of the body or by increasing body temperature in general. Overheating may occur from:

- Wearing snug-fitting briefs or other tight clothing
- Frequent use of hot tubs, saunas, or jacuzzis
- Heavy exercise
- Working in certain jobs that involve excessive heat like factory work near a furnace

Lose Excess Weight. Being overweight can adversely affect sperm production because the excess weight can cause the body to have greater contact with the scrotum, increasing body temperature. Being overweight can also signify a hormonal problem or diabetes, which can decrease sperm production.

Recover Fully from Infections or Illnesses That Involve Fever. Fever usually causes the entire body to heat up, thus reducing sperm count and quality.

Reduce Exposure to Harmful Work or Recreational Environments. Such environments may involve reproductive hazards such as environmental toxins like hazardous chemicals or exposure to radiation that can affect fertility (see the "Male Reproductive Hazards" chart in Chapter 1).

What You Can Do

Gain or Lose Weight. Being over- or underweight can also affect a woman's ability to conceive.

Being severely underweight affects menstruation and can even stop ovulation and menstrual periods. Being underweight from exercising a lot can also affect your fertility. Let your OB provider know if you think you have an eating disorder such as anorexia or bulimia.

If you're overweight, you may have a problem with your endocrine system. This system produces the hormones of your body and can affect the hormones of ovulation.

When to Seek Help

If you have concerns about becoming pregnant, you should schedule an appointment with your OB/GYN provider. He or she may tell you to relax and give it more time, depending upon your medical history, your age, and the amount of time you and your partner have been trying to get pregnant.

If you're under 35, he or she may recommend that you try for a year to get pregnant before seeking further medical advice and assistance.

If you're over 35, your OB/GYN provider will probably suggest that both of you be evaluated for infertility after six months of trying unsuccessfully to conceive. Age is a critical factor for fertility, especially for females.

Factors That May Require the Help of a Professional

The following may be factors affecting your ability to conceive. Many of them can be resolved, enabling you to have a baby:

- Not having regular menstrual periods
- Having had three or more miscarriages

- If either you or your partner had a fertility problem with an earlier relationship
- If either you or your partner had certain infections that can affect fertility, such as:
  - Adult males who have had mumps as a teenager or prostate infection
  - Adult females who have had pelvic inflammatory disease (PID)
  - Adult females who have had a chlamydia or gonorrhea infection that affected the fallopian tubes

Be assured that even if you have one or more of these factors in your health history, there are many things that can be done to improve your chances of conceiving. Implementing these measures requires the expertise of your OB Provider and possibly a reproductive endocrinologist.

What, Not Who, Causes Infertility

There are many reasons why a couple might have problems with getting pregnant. If you're beginning to think that you, as a couple, are having an infertility problem, it is important to think in terms of *what*, not who, is causing the problem. You must leave the issue of blame behind. It's not productive for either member of the couple to think of infertility as "your problem, not mine." Work together as a couple, support one another, try consciously to have the best possible communication with each other. Be willing to talk about your feelings, your fears, your stress, and your frustration.

Medical Evaluation

The first step to discovering why you aren't getting pregnant is to see an OB/GYN provider or a reproductive endocrinologist for an evaluation. This provider will thoroughly review both of your medical histories. There will be lots of questions, some very intimate and personal. Remind yourself that the answers to these questions may provide a clue to treat your cause of infertility. Most providers who work with fertility issues are sensitive to your feelings and will be careful and professional.

Female Evaluation for Infertility

The initial health assessment includes a complete physical examination, a pap smear, and pelvic exam. You will be asked to fill out a detailed questionnaire about your menstruation patterns—frequency or regularity, amount of flow, degree of pain, any previous pregnancies, the possibility of STDs, and your method of birth control. You'll have an assessment of your general health, and blood will be taken for hormone testing to see if you are producing eggs. Most infertility problems are caused by ovarian dysfunction.

Tests for Infertility Might Include

- A blood test for detecting the presence of the hormone progesterone and thyroid function. Blood tests also establish that your other hormones are within normal limits, and provide a measurement of your general health.
- An endometrial biopsy to examine cells from the lining of your uterus for evidence that your body has prepared for ovulation by thickening the uterine lining, and if or when ovulation has occurred. For this procedure, a small, flexible, plastic tube is inserted through your vagina and cervix into the uterus to scrape off a few cells of the endometrium.
- Your doctor may examine your uterus, ovaries, and fallopian tubes for signs of damage, blockage, or abnormalities using ultrasound, an X ray, or both.

There are several avenues to explore to find out why you might be having difficulty conceiving. Your doctor must determine if you're having problems with any one or a combination of the following factors:

- Maturing eggs (hormonal or genetic problem)
- Ovulating (hormonal problem)
- A blockage that prevents a fertilized egg from leaving the fallopian tube (structural problem)
- Inability of the egg to implant in the lining of the uterus (hormonal or structural problem)

Infertility from Hormonal Problems

Normal hormone function is critical to fertility. The most common disruption of normal hormonal function is simply aging. The frequently talked about "biological clock" is very real.

Over time, the function of the ovaries changes. At puberty, when ovulation and menstruation begins, you have about 300,000 eggs. One egg is ripened and released from an ovary each month. Also each month, 500 or more eggs disintegrate within the ovary, never to ripen or be released for possible fertilization. Losing about 500 eggs a month means your egg supply is depleting by leaps and bounds.[4] Even though your eggs are depleting, you probably do have eggs. They can be stimulated with medication to ripen and release from the ovaries. This is called "ovulation induction." By the end of your reproductive years, usually when a person is in her mid-forties, relatively few eggs are left and many have genetic abnormalities. Having an aging reproductive system affects the other steps needed to produce a baby.

As your ovaries become more sluggish and your eggs age, levels of FSH and LH increase and ovarian estrogen declines. Over time, the ovaries become increasingly more resistant to FSH and LH stimulation. Without appropriate ovarian response (i.e., increased estrogen production) to these hormones, an egg will fail to mature and you may not ovulate consistently on a monthly basis. But larger amounts of FSH and LH may not produce a ripened egg. When the ovaries can't or don't respond to the FSH and LH, estrogen and progesterone levels also decrease. This limits the chances for a pregnancy because these hormones are critical to being able to successfully develop the lining of the uterus, where the embryo must implant.

Ovulation Induction

The medications used for ovulation induction are often referred to as fertility drugs. They work by stimulating the ovaries to ripen and release eggs.

- The most commonly prescribed medication is *clomiphene citrate*. This pill-form medication stimulates the release of GnRH or the gonadotropin-releasing hormone, which directs the pituitary gland to produce more FSH and LH.
- Newer medications are synthetic FSH or combinations of FSH and LH. These are referred to as gonadotropin (GTN) and are prescribed for women who obtain no results with clomiphene. It is injected daily for about 5–7 days by a shot you give yourself or it can be given by your partner.
- Human chorionic gonadotropin (hCG) is a one-time only injection administered about 24 hours after the last dose of clomiphene citrate or gonadotropin. It stimulates the ovary to release the matured egg.

Results from these treatments are very good if the cause of infertility is ovarian dysfunction. Over three-quarters of those women who take medication to induce ovulation begin ovulating. Half of the women who have difficulty getting pregnant because of ovarian dysfunction become pregnant within six months of trying the above treatments, if there are no other obstacles to conception.[5]

Risks from Ovulation Induction

The medications used to treat infertility resulting from ovarian dysfunction have been very successful. However, they are not without some risks. The most common risk is the increased chance of having a multiple gestation, meaning having more than one baby in one pregnancy—twins, triplets, or more.

Aside from the shock of learning that you may be raising several babies at once, carrying multiples makes a pregnancy high-risk, even if it's "just twins." See Chapter 4 for the risk of preterm labor and Chapter 10 about having twins or other multiples. Fortunately, careful monitoring by specialists in ovulation induction has proven effective in reducing the number of pregnancies with multiple gestations.

Another health risk of fertility medication is ovarian hyperstimulation syndrome. That is, the hormones used to stimulate the production and release of an egg can also cause ovaries to enlarge significantly with extra fluid. This fluid is transferred to the abdomen, creating a condition called *ascities*. Ovarian hyperstimulation syndrome and the resulting ascities usually are treated with bedrest or hospitalization. Fortunately, this condition is not common.

Other Factors

Changes in Eggs That Occur with Age. Your eggs were created while you were a fetus inside your mother's uterus. As you age, your remaining eggs become less fertile because of changes that take place over time. They may carry genetic disorders. Eggs with genetic disorders are less likely to become fertilized. If they are fertilized, the embryos are more likely to be aborted, resulting in miscarriage. If you're ovulating but having difficulty becoming pregnant, your OB/GYN provider may suggest genetic testing and counseling to discover if aging eggs are the source of your fertility problem.

Polycystic Ovarian Syndrome. Your OB/GYN provider may suspect that PCOS is the cause of your infertility if you have irregular or absent menstruation, difficulty maintaining ideal weight, facial hair growth, and acne. Some women with PCOS are unable to convert glucose normally, which can be a sign of future diabetes. PCOS occurs when there is a hormonal imbalance between FSH, LH, estrogen, and testosterone. Multiple follicular cysts are present within the ovaries and insufficient FSH may suppress ovulation. Elevations in the male type androgen testosterone may also reduce ovulation, but you can become pregnant with this condition. Your OB/GYN provider will work with you to regulate your weight and may prescribe hormone medication for ovulation induction.

Unknown Ovarian Dysfunction. Your OB/GYN may not be able to determine why you are not ovulating, only that you are not.

Female Structural Problems

If you're producing eggs and ovulating, but are not conceiving, your OB/GYN provider may look for signs of structural blockage, particularly of the fallopian tubes, as the cause of your infertility. Endometriosis, pelvic inflammatory disease (PID), reversed tubal ligation, or scarring from previous unrelated abdominal surgery might be causing the blockage. If you have any of these problems, you are not alone. One-third of infertility cases are caused by blockage of the fallopian tubes.[6] Fortunately, physicians specializing in fertility have several options for treating this kind of infertility. There are several possible causes of blocked fallopian tubes.

Endometriosis

In endometriosis, tissue from the lining of your uterus, the endometrium, which sheds every month as part of a woman's normal menstrual flow, does not leave the body through normal menstrual flow. Instead, it backs up into the abdominal cavity and remains there to start lesions. These lesions are also called implants, nodules, or growths.

At the sites where the endometrial tissue adheres, such as the bowel, fallopian tubes, ovaries, uterus, or bladder, the tissue continues to respond to reproductive hormones. Each month, the tissue builds up and then shed or bleeds. This causes inflammation, swelling, and eventually scarring of the surrounding tissue. When this process occurs in the fallopian tubes, the scarred tissue can cause blockage of the tubes, and when this occurs in the uterus, it can prevent a fertilized egg from implanting.

Symptoms of endometriosis include pain during or after sexual activity, severe menstrual cramps, and occasional abdominal pain even when menstruation is not occurring.

Endometriosis can be both a hormonal and structural problem. Your OB provider may recommend hormone treatments that suppress your menstrual cycle and prevent the endometrial lesions from building up. After a period of several months, your provider will then take you off hormone treatment, recommending that you try to conceive immediately. If this does not work or is not an option, the OB provider may recommend removal of the endometrial lesions with a surgical procedure.

Though endometriosis that leads to extensive scarring of the reproductive organs is one of the major causes of infertility, mild endometriosis can often be treated with surgery and medication. And many women with endometriosis, which may or may not require treatment, will be able to conceive.[7]

Pelvic Inflammatory Disease

The primary cause of PID is a severe infection in your fallopian tubes, and sometimes the uterus. The infection causes inflammation and, as a result, leads to scarring of the tissue. As with endometriosis, the scarred tissue cannot perform normally. If the fallopian tubes are blocked, eggs may be prevented from getting into the tube to be fertilized or, once fertilized, the embryo can't get out of the tube to implant in the uterus.

PID is diagnosed by a physical exam, blood tests, ultrasound, and an investigative procedure called *laparoscopy*, which will show whether there are swollen tubes or if there's scarring. Some women are thought to have gotten PID from using an older version of the IUD or from exposure to sexually transmitted diseases like gonorrhea and chlamydia. Sometimes no cause can be determined.

While PID is a serious disease that can cause difficulty with getting pregnant, it may be possible to conceive a baby even if you have it. Only one fallopian tube needs to function properly in order for conception to occur. If tube blockage is the infertility problem, your OB provider will try to correct it in one of two ways. Sometimes the tubes can be opened during the initial examination of these areas; other times surgery is needed to open up or repair the tubes.

Fibroids

Fibroids, also called *myomas* or *leiomyomas*, are noncancerous tumors of uterine muscle tissue. They grow in or on the outside of the uterus and, more rarely, in the cervix. What causes a fibroid is unclear, but they often grow larger during pregnancy and then shrink after menopause, indicating their link with changing levels of estrogen.

Fibroids are diagnosed using examination, ultrasound, and some types of X-ray procedures. Most fibroids develop in women in their 30s and 40s. Usually there are no symptoms and the fibroids require no treatment. Noticeable symptoms include excessive bleeding during menstruation, pain, and abdominal or bladder pressure.

Having fibroids is very common, but only 2 to 3 percent of all women with fibroids have difficulty becoming pregnant because of them.[8]

Fertility may be affected by fibroids in several ways. The fibroid may:

- Alter the endometrium and make it difficult for the embryo to implant
- Take up space in the uterine cavity where the embryo is trying to implant
- Be located near a fallopian tube and compress it so that the egg and sperm cannot pass through

While fibroids do not often cause infertility, they can be an important factor in later stages of pregnancy (see Chapter 11).

Abnormal Shape of Reproductive Tract Organs

Your doctor may discover that you have an abnormally formed uterus or that other organs of the reproductive tract may be interfering with conception. There are a number of surgical options to correct these abnormalities.

Male Fertility Problems

When a couple is having trouble getting pregnant, both the man and woman must be examined and evaluated. A reproductive endocrinologist or an andrologist—a specialist in male infertility—tries to determine whether your partner's sperm are healthy, well-formed, mobile, and numerous, and that the seminal fluid is normal. If any of these characteristics are not normal, additional tests may reveal infections, hormonal imbalances, or other problems. Most of the problems are correctable, enabling you both to continue pursuing having a baby.

Male fertility evaluation begins with a semen analysis. Your partner will be given a sterile specimen cup and will be asked to step into a private room supplied with a few magazines. He will need to masturbate until he gets semen into the cup. Male sperm must be analyzed to see if they are healthy and if there are enough sperm in the semen. Although it is not ideal, if your partner is uncomfortable with masturbating or is prohibited from doing it for religious reasons, a sample may also be obtained by sending you both home and letting him try to get a sample after intercourse by withdrawing before ejaculation, or by using a laboratory-approved condom. Your partner must follow special instructions to ensure that he gets as uncontaminated a sample as possible. The withdrawal method of collection can result in a smaller sample or one that may be contaminated by vaginal bacteria.

Once collected and sent to the lab, the semen analysis begins. The sperm are examined for number, shape, movement, and presence of infection. Well-shaped, motile sperm are a good indicator of male fertility.

Low Sperm Count and Ability to Ejaculate

Sometimes the specialist finds only a few sperm in the sample. Few sperm or a low sperm count does not necessarily prevent fertilization.

Sperm count is the number of active sperm in a certain amount of semen and normal is usually 20 to 150 million sperm per milliliter.[9] However, conception can and does occur with far fewer sperm. If the sperm count is low, the andrologist, using X-ray or ultrasound analysis, looks at the reproductive structure—to see if something is preventing the sperm from leaving the testes and being ejaculated.

Structural injury to the vas deferens—which are the ducts, or tubes, that lead from the testes to the penis and are necessary for ejaculation of sperm—is the most common cause of low sperm count. The vas deferens may have been blocked on purpose with male sterilization—a vasectomy, or by previous unrelated surgery. Or they may have been blocked by disease, sexually transmitted or otherwise. In some cases the andrologist may be able to open the blockage during the diagnosis. In others, microsurgery may be successful in repairing the blocked vas deferens.

Sometimes the sperm appear quite normal except that they don't move. If that proves to be the circumstance, the specialist may want to extract a sample of sperm directly from the testes to see if sperm from there can move normally. Some men have nonfunctioning sperm in their ejaculate but live sperm in their testes. This is thought to be caused by chemicals in the seminal fluid that are not usually harmful but, for unknown reasons, are harmful in certain cases.

Having abundant sperm is not the most important factor in male infertility. Equally important factors are motility, or the ability of the sperm to move, and the ability of the sperm to penetrate the egg. The sperm must be able to wriggle forward and break through the *zona*, or covering, of the egg. Sperm that have been ejaculated go through the *acrosome*, or egg-penetrating, reaction once inside the female reproductive system. The sperm pick up speed, a process called *capacitation*, and release digestive enzymes from the acrosome cap at the top or "head" of the sperm. The digestive enzymes allow sperm to get through the egg covering and fertilize the egg.

Treating the Inability to Ejaculate. Some men are not able to ejaculate. Inability to ejaculate can be caused by problems such as diabetes, surgery on the prostate gland or urethra, blood pressure or other medications, spinal cord injury, cancer treatment, or impotence. For some of these cases, reproductive specialists can use electrical stimulation to cause an ejaculation or surgical removal of the sperm.

Treating Low Sperm Count. As mentioned previously, absence of sperm or low sperm count may be due to a variety of factors including abnormalities of the semen, testicular structural blockage that cannot be repaired, hormonal imbalance, inability to ejaculate, or inability of the sperm to penetrate the egg and fertilize it. Fertilization requires a series of chemical reactions that allow one sperm to penetrate one egg cell. If that does not happen, a single sperm can be collected from the semen or from the testes and injected directly into each mature egg to produce embryos. This is one kind of assisted reproductive technology, which we will discuss next.

Assisted Reproductive Technologies

Even after thorough, examination and treatment, you still may not be able to conceive. When there is a medical indication, your OB provider or fertility specialist may suggest that advanced fertility treatment, called Assisted Reproductive Technologies (ART) is needed.

These technologies use highly technical procedures and medical expertise to enable couples to have a baby that is biologically theirs. In cases of more complicated infertility problems, such as poor egg or sperm quality, these technologies can be used to help couples conceive even when they might have thought it would not be possible.

ART enables many couples to have children when every other "natural" method has failed. These technologies are truly miraculous. If your OB provider or fertility specialist has recommended that you consider this option in your quest to have a baby, he or she will be able to refer you to organizations dedicated to helping couples have babies with these technologies. These organizations will provide you with lots of up-to-date material to help you understand this next step.

The Basics of In Vitro Fertilization

Assisted reproductive technologies are changing so rapidly that current information is soon out of date. The core technology, however, remains the same and is based on *in vitro fertilization*.

If you're undergoing IVF, you will take ovulation induction medication to stimulate your ovaries to ripen several eggs and to prepare your endometrium for implantation. When the eggs have ripened, they're surgically removed. Your partner produces sperm, either with ejaculation or through surgical extraction from the testes. Eggs and sperm are mixed in a petri dish, or sperm are directly injected into several eggs. The mixture is watched under a microscope for evidence of fertilization.

Because several eggs and several sperm are together, you can have more than one embryo develop. After several days about two to five embryos(depending on your age) will be selected, placed in a catheter, and injected into your uterus by way of your vagina. Any extras can be frozen for possible later use if this attempt at pregnancy fails or if an additional later pregnancy is desired. Two weeks after the embryos have been placed in the uterus, a pregnancy blood test will be performed to determine if any of the embryos implanted successfully in the uterine wall. A definitive "You are pregnant!" requires three more weeks, when the implanted embryos can be seen by ultrasound.

ART has become quite successful. Currently about one quarter of couples that try ART deliver a baby or babies. Because so many women in their late 40s and 50s have successfully gotten pregnant either using IVF or donor egg programs, the Centers for Disease Control has begun keeping statistical track of this brand new category of mothers.

Getting Pregnant

Getting pregnant can be "a walk in the park" or "an uphill battle," and everything in between. However you become pregnant, it is the obvious next step in your journey. Our wish for you is that it will be a joyful union and a wonderful start of a new life.

3

Congratulations, You're Pregnant! Now What?

 Sonia's Journal (two months pregnant)

Dear Journal,

It's been a rough week. One minute I'm on top of the world and the next I'm scared. I have no energy, and when I don't feel tired, I feel sick to my stomach. I tried to talk to Brian about it, but he shrugged his shoulders helplessly. I know this "morning sickness" is supposed to only last for a month or two, but when I am in the middle of it, I feel like I can't bear it another minute. I didn't realize it would feel so awful. On the other hand, I got a "pregnancy" magazine in the mail today and found myself falling in love with all the pictures of babies. I can hardly wait to hold my baby in my arms. When I think about how great it's going to be, I know I can get through this first rough patch.

Whether you're pregnant for the first or the fourth time, you'll most likely feel a spectrum of emotions, from surprise to joy and fear. If you're a "first-timer," you may experience a "fear of the unknown," although even an experienced mother may feel some apprehension, especially if she encountered some unexpected problem in earlier pregnancies. However, along with nervousness comes the excitement of actually carrying another "being" inside your body. Your baby is growing inside of you—you're going to be a mother!

During the next nine months, you'll undergo many physical changes and emotional adjustments. Initially, you may find yourself concentrating on whatever is happening in the present, instead of thinking about the future. The early symptoms of pregnancy, such as nausea or fatigue, will hold a lot of your attention, along with beginning to accept the idea that you really are pregnant. Even later in the pregnancy, after most of the physical changes have already occurred, you'll probably still focus on what's currently happening to your body and the emotions accompanying those changes.

Why the Mixed Feelings?

The spectrum of moods you experience while pregnant are in part due to your hormones. They're helping your body make dramatic changes. Different hormone levels can make you moody, quickly switching between highs and lows. The circumstances surrounding your pregnancy can also affect how you feel. Whether you were planning the pregnancy or not, how your partner feels about it and your own feelings about whether you can financially afford a child or are ready to be pregnant and have a baby are considerations that can affect your mood.

Developing a positive outlook is the first step to ensuring a healthy birth. Along with being physically prepared, you also need to be mentally and emotionally prepared. Even if you have fears and mixed feelings about your pregnancy, if you take care of yourself and develop a strong partnership with an OB provider, you'll be off to a good start.

An expectant mother's motivation during her pregnancy can be a critical component in the health of her unborn child. Some unexpected events in pregnancy cannot be controlled, but your attitude and willingness to work with your OB provider can help you protect your health and the health of your baby.

To cope with the range of emotions you may be feeling, and to improve your sense of well-being, consider writing down your thoughts about your pregnancy and communicating them with your husband or partner. Talk with friends or family members who have children. They'll probably tell you they felt similarly in the beginning of their pregnancies. Remind yourself that while this is exciting, it's also new, and anything new usually includes some trepidation. If you feel you're having an unusual level of anxiety about your pregnancy, talk with your OB provider. He or she can help set your mind at ease or recommend a counselor who can work with you to try to alleviate your anxieties.

TRY THIS: MAKE A PREGNANCY NOTEBOOK

This is a great time to start a pregnancy notebook. You can keep track of your questions for your OB provider and of important changes in your pregnancy, along with recording your thoughts and feelings as your baby grows inside you. Tape a calendar with the future months of your pregnancy in the notebook to keep track of exactly how many weeks pregnant you are.

Start at the back of the notebook, writing *Week 40* on the day your baby is due to be born, and count back each week, labeling each day of the previous week with the gestational age. If you're due May 28 on a Thursday, the exact day or the week before that is Thursday May 21. Mark this page *Week 39*, mark the page before this, Thursday May 14, *Week 38*, and so forth. Your OB provider will often refer to how many weeks along you are. This will help you keep your own record of your pregnancy.

Sample notebook entry:

Thursday, February 14

Week 12

10:00 a.m. prenatal appointment

Must tell nurse practitioner that the nausea is better.

We have decided to have amniocentesis. Find out how to schedule this.

Ask if my trip to Puerto Rico in Week 20 is okay.

Pick up Brian's Valentine's present after work.

First Steps

Congratulations, you're going to be a mother! Be happy—be thrilled! The first thing to do is take a deep breath, smile, and call to make an appointment with your OB provider as soon as possible. The medical professional you choose will guide you through this pregnancy. (For more guidance on which kind of obstetric provider you'd like for your pregnancy, see Chapter 1.)

You will learn a lot about your pregnancy at each visit, so it's important to make your medical appointments a priority. It's your job to activate your involvement with your medical team. Consider bringing a list of questions to discuss with your doctor or midwife during your office visit, such as what may happen during the phases of pregnancy and when you should call about problems.

The Importance of Early Prenatal Care

Prenatal visits monitor the health of you and your baby, and prepare you for the changes—both physical and emotional—of pregnancy. Regular prenatal visits also allow your obstetrics provider to monitor the growth of your baby. For most of your pregnancy, the prenatal visits will be monthly. They will give you an opportunity to share both your excitement and any concern about how your body is changing with medical professionals whose primary aim is to help you have a great pregnancy and birth experience.

On your initial visit, your chosen obstetrics professional will confirm the pregnancy and assess your general and reproductive health. He or she will administer a blood test to determine your blood type and learn more about your health. This test may also screen for genetic disorders and look for the presence of anemia or sexually transmitted diseases.

On subsequent visits, your doctor will measure your vital signs—such as blood pressure and pulse to determine how your body is responding to the pregnancy. Regular urine tests are administered in order to look for abnormal levels of sugar and protein, since this could indicate complications such as diabetes and high blood pressure. With prenatal visits, any potential problems can be detected early on, making it easier for them to be corrected before they make your pregnancy difficult for you or your baby.

SARA'S STORY

Sara was 24 weeks pregnant and due for a scheduled prenatal checkup but was also under a deadline at work. Feeling fine she was tempted to reschedule her appointment for later in the week, but decided to keep the scheduled appointment. During the checkup, the nurse midwife had noticed that Sara's blood pressure was higher than normal. High blood pressure in pregnant women can harm both the mother and the baby. The midwife consulted with her physician, and Sara was given medication and asked to increase her rest to treat her high blood pressure. Early intervention by the nurse midwife and doctor helped detect Sara's problem. Her blood pressure was under control throughout the rest of the pregnancy and she delivered a healthy baby.

Things You Can Do for a Healthy Pregnancy

Your baby is completely dependent on you to provide the best environment for him or her to grow. Eating healthy food and taking care of your body will make your womb a safe place for your child. Eating healthy food and exercising will also benefit you, giving you the vitality and good health you need to enjoy your pregnancy.

Eating Right

For healthiest pregnancy eating, follow the rules of the USDA's Food Guide Pyramid. That means eating foods high in protein and complex carbohydrates and low in fat and sugar. If you're a vegetarian and/or do not eat dairy products or meat, you need to talk to your doctor to make sure you're getting enough B-12, a vitamin found only in meat and milk. You will also want to boost your consumption of foods that are high in calcium, iron, and fiber.

TRY THIS

Take a sheet of paper and write down what you ate yesterday. Include beverages, snacks, and anything you spread on your foods or used to cook your food. Also include how much you ate; for instance, *two slices of toast*, or *one eight-ounce bag of chips*. Remember to count the number of caffeinated products, like soda, coffee, or tea. (These do not count toward your total water intake.) Next, using the U.S. Department of Agriculture's Food Guide Pyramid (Figure 3-1), label the items by their food group. Note approximately how much of each food group you consumed. How did you do? Did you follow the pyramid? Are you truly eating as well or as badly as you thought? Do you have ideas about how you can improve?

Food Guide Pyramid
A Guide to Daily Food Choices for Pregnant Women

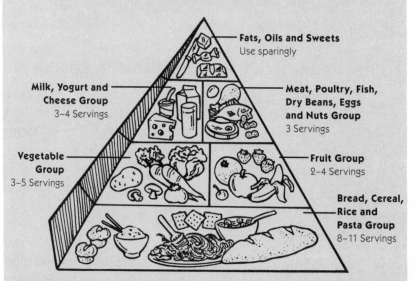

Fats, Oils and Sweets
Use sparingly

Milk, Yogurt and Cheese Group
3–4 Servings

Meat, Poultry, Fish, Dry Beans, Eggs and Nuts Group
3 Servings

Vegetable Group
3–5 Servings

Fruit Group
2–4 Servings

Bread, Cereal, Rice and Pasta Group
8–11 Servings

FIGURE 3-1   The Food Pyramid: USDA-recommended daily food choices for pregnant women.

Source: U.S. Dept. of Agriculture.

Increase Calcium

Everyone needs calcium to build and replenish bones and muscles. Calcium is also important to your baby's development in utero. All women need calcium throughout their lives but many find it hard to take in enough. Women of childbearing age should have about 1000 milligrams. of calcium daily, whether they're pregnant or not.

The easiest way to add calcium to your diet is to increase your consumption of dairy products. To minimize fat intake, drink skim or low-fat milk and eat low-fat cheeses and yogurts. If you are lactose intolerant or allergic to dairy, salmon and sardines are good sources of calcium. If you follow a vegetarian diet that does not include dairy, increase your consumption of dark green leafy vegetables such as collard greens, turnip greens, and kale, and include more legumes such as dried beans and peas.

Other sources for calcium include nuts and seeds, cooked rhubarb, acorn squash, and tofu. Spinach, while high in calcium, also contains oxalic acid, which may inhibit the body's ability to absorb the calcium. If you feel you don't take in enough calcium daily, you should ask your OB provider about taking supplements such as calcium citrate or carbonate.

Increase Iron

Iron is important in the formation of new blood cells for both mother and baby and to prevent anemia in the mother. The recommended minimum daily allowance for women who are not pregnant is 15 milligrams. For pregnant women the RDA doubles to 30 milligrams!

Beef liver, clams, oysters, roast beef, hamburger, sardines, canned tuna, ham, chicken, eggs, almonds, and peanut butter are good sources of iron. Many commercial cereals have been fortified with vitamins and minerals, including iron. Fruits high in iron are dried apricots, raisins, prunes, and prune juice. Vegetables high in iron include spinach, potatoes, peas, acorn squash, brussels sprouts, dandelion greens, broccoli, lima beans, and tomato juice. Eating foods high in vitamin C at the same time as eating foods high in iron will help your body absorb more iron.

Increase Fiber

Fiber, also known as "roughage" or "bulk," is the indigestible part of plants. It's a good idea to start increasing the level of fiber in your food early in your pregnancy because a sudden increase can cause gas and other abdominal distress.

Adding fiber to your diet will speed the passage of waste matter, including some toxins, through your digestive tract. This will be especially important later in your pregnancy, when the baby's size begins to put pressure on your intestines while slowing their ability to eliminate waste. Without enough roughage, you may become constipated and develop hemorrhoids toward the end of your pregnancy. Hemorrhoids are swollen veins that are pushed out of the rectum when you strain to have a bowel movement. They are often itchy and painful.

Sources of fiber include fruits, vegetables, whole grains, nuts, and seeds. The National Cancer Institute recommends that everyone—pregnant or not—take in 20 to 35 grams of fiber daily. If you were to eat a bowl of bran cereal, a half cup of beans, two fruits, and one vegetable a day, you would be adding about 22 grams of fiber to your diet.

Increase Water

Drink eight glasses of water per day. This extra fluid is needed to increase your blood volume. Fluids also help prevent constipation and flush waste materials from the body more quickly. Having sufficient water in your system can improve your metabolism. Later in your pregnancy drinking enough fluids will prevent dehydration, which can lead to preterm labor contractions. Drinking more water also helps your kidneys—which are working for two—wash salts and waste out of your system. Reducing salts may also help prevent swelling in your hands and feet.

Decrease Harmful Foods

You want to maximize the value of the nutritious foods you're adding to your pregnancy diet, and caffeine blocks the body's ability to absorb and utilize calcium and iron. So drink less than two cups of caffeinated beverages a day. Caffeine also acts as a stimulant and may prevent you from getting needed rest, and it's a diuretic—removing fluids from the system—and therefore may cause dehydration.

If you feel it's too difficult to eliminate that afternoon soda or cup of coffee, try substituting this habit with a quick walk around the block. A little stretching of your muscles may give you the lift you're used to getting from caffeine, as well as allow you a few moments to reflect on how well you're coming along in your pregnancy.

Contact your local health department to learn about local warnings about fish. *Limit your consumption of freshwater fish and shoreline dwelling fish* if they have high levels of pesticides or other toxins. Ocean fish that live far offshore seem to be the safest, except for swordfish and tuna, which can contain high levels of methyl mercury. Other fish that may contain a significant amount of contaminants include striped bass, bluefish, catfish, and carp. *Avoid raw milk and raw eggs.* Raw milk has not been pasteurized to remove harmful microbes. Raw eggs, sometimes used in dishes such as Caesar salad, may contain the microbe salmonella, which can make you very sick. Raw shellfish and sushi can also contain microbes that will make you sick to your stomach. Vomiting and bouts of diarrhea are not only unpleasant, they can make you dangerously dehydrated. Dehydration is a danger at any time but especially during pregnancy. Most institutions serving food have changed their recipes to avoid raw egg, but it doesn't hurt to confirm this when you are dining out.

Avoid sugar and fat substitutes. Foods made with chemical substitutes may be harmful. Try to eat foods that are naturally sweetened and naturally low-fat, such as fruit. Use your pregnancy and your desire to make the best choices for your baby as a reason for making lifelong beneficial changes in your diet by eliminating low or no-cal processed food and beverages. Staying healthy during pregnancy helps you give your baby a healthy foundation.

Taking Vitamins

You may be currently taking a multivitamin or supplements from a health food store. It's very important to let your OB provider know what you've been taking even if you think that the vitamins and/or supplements are harmless. Some natural herbs and vitamins can cause problems in pregnancy. In most cases, your doctor will ask you to replace any vitamins you're currently taking with a prescription prenatal vitamin. This will supply everything your baby needs for its development, and it will maintain your health as well.

Pregnancy Weight Gain

Everyone wants to know how much weight they'll gain during pregnancy. Most doctors and midwives recommend that you increase your daily calorie intake during pregnancy by 300 calories. This will vary depending on your prepregnancy weight.

Women at a normal weight at the start of their pregnancies should gain about 25 to 35 pounds. Women who are underweight can gain more, and overweight women should of course gain less. (See Chapter 1 to calculate your body mass index.) You will be weighed during each prenatal visit to make sure you're on track for your recommended weight gain.

Exercising During Pregnancy

You're probably familiar with the health benefits of exercise, for everyone. Exercise is also very important during pregnancy. However, *the goal of exercise in pregnancy should not be to lose weight.*

Exercise has three components: weight training, stretching, and aerobic. The most important of these three before and during early pregnancy is aerobic, and the primary purpose is to strengthen your heart so that at rest it does not have to beat as quickly to pump blood through your system. With aerobic exercise, your heart becomes more efficient, which has a number of benefits for a healthy pregnancy.

For one thing, regular exercise will make you feel more energetic and may make you feel emotionally better by leveling out erratic moods. For another, it will help you sleep more soundly and improve muscle tone and posture. Exercise will also benefit your pregnancy by reducing backaches and minimizing constipation and bloating. And finally, it will give you the stamina to manage the work of childbirth. Use caution when doing aerobic exercise so as not to fall.

There are specific and normal pregnancy changes in your body that will affect how exercise feels to you. The hormones of pregnancy will loosen your joints and make them more relaxed. Also, because your body's blood volume is increasing and you're carrying more weight, you'll also have an increased heart rate. These changes may necessitate some adjustments in your form of exercise. For instance, you will be at maximum blood volume at Week 25 of pregnancy, and it's important then not to drop your head below your heart during exercise because greater blood volume means your blood is not circulating as quickly—you may feel light-headed.

Stretching exercises throughout pregnancy are beneficial, but as with any exercise you must be careful to stretch only after warming up your muscles, and even then to stretch only to the point of feeling tension and not pulling. Pregnancy will also bring an altered sense of balance: You may not feel as steady on your feet at times. Many OB providers will tell you it's okay to continue weight-training if you've been doing it all along. Keep safety techniques in mind and remember to exhale when lifting. If you hold your breath, your blood pressure goes up, and you want to avoid this during pregnancy. In short, most kinds of exercise are in fact okay during pregnancy, but try to avoid exercise that's particularly bouncy or jarring. And after the 20th week of pregnancy you should not do exercises that require you to lie flat on your back, since this reduces blood flow to the uterus. Of course, you should also consider stopping activities that could lead to falls and injuries, such as mountain biking.

Getting Started

Ideally, you had an exercise program in place before you became pregnant. If you didn't exercise regularly before, you can begin now. As noted in the previous section, pregnancy will bring you all kinds of new physical sensations. If you start an exercise regimen early in the pregnancy, you'll be better able to sort out what is a result of exercise and what is a consequence of being pregnant.

Enrolling in an exercise for pregnancy class where the instructor can monitor your response may be your best bet. Walking is also a fine exercise for your heart and whole body. For safety and companionship, get someone to go with you. A 20-minute walk three times a week will strengthen your heart and prepare you for the work of carrying your baby late in the pregnancy, and it will help you during labor.

Other than pregnancy exercise classes and walking, swimming and yoga are considered good kinds of exercise for pregnant women. With all kinds of exercise, remember to keep well hydrated and include a warmup and cool-down period. To do these, begin with a few stretches and by walking slowly for a few minutes, and do the same at the end of exercising. If you already exercise regularly and are now pregnant, get advice from your doctor or midwife about continuing your form and amount of exercise throughout the pregnancy. Some complications of pregnancy can make exercising unwise. Again, follow the directions of your OB provider.

Mapping Out Your Pregnancy

Now that you have an idea concerning some of the healthy lifestyle actions you'll want to take to protect your baby and yourself while pregnant, let's take a look at the specific stages of your pregnancy. The three sections of your journey are referred to in medical terminology as the three trimesters. Each trimester lasts three months—making up the nine months (or 40 weeks) of pregnancy. Knowing what to expect in each trimester will prepare you for a better experience of the pregnancy journey.

Your First Trimester

Congratulations, you're about to start your journey through pregnancy! The end of the journey may seem very far away, but your pregnancy will go by very quickly and you'll be cuddling your baby before you know it!

What You Can Expect

The first few weeks of the first trimester of pregnancy are very exciting because, while you are pregnant, you may have few physical signs.

Truly a miracle! You may wonder if anyone can tell you're pregnant. You might want to tell everyone you meet, but at the same time, barely believe it yourself. Some women get anxious and worry that if they tell everyone right away this will jinx their condition. This is a normal fear. It's usually a sign that you're experiencing the desire to protect your pregnancy and your baby.

TRY THIS

Write a Letter to Your Child

- Describe how you feel at this point in your pregnancy.
- Retell how you were told that you were pregnant and what you first said.
- Describe how your partner reacted when he or she first heard the news.
- Write promises to yourself to take one day at a time and to try to be good to yourself and your baby for the next nine months. Promise you will ask for help when you need it.

The first trimester lasts till Week 13. These are the first, second, and third months of your pregnancy. Many women don't know they are pregnant until they're halfway through this first trimester, and other than realizing their period is late, they don't have any of the usual symptoms of early pregnancy.

Even though you may not feel any different, your body is going through incredible changes. These changes will eventually cause some early symptoms of pregnancy, which can be unpleasant but are normal. While being tired and/or nauseous is no fun, it does make your pregnancy very real, and such a confirmation can add to your excitement. Happily, these early discomforts will go away over time or can be managed with some modification in your daily routine.

The early symptoms of pregnancy include:

- *Fatigue.* You may feel very tired throughout the day or at times feel you have never experienced such fatigue before. You may crave a nap each day. The fatigue is caused by the rapid growth of your uterus and your baby, both demanding energy from your body.

Tip: Plan for this rest time. Don't fight the urge for a nap. Schedule time in your day just to rest. Even if you don't sleep, just put your feet up and drink some water. You'll feel better, less tired, and perhaps less moody.

- *Breast Tenderness.* Your breast tissue will swell in response to the buildup of hormones in your body, specifically increased estrogen. This hormone also helps thicken the lining of the uterus, which nourishes your baby in the early part of pregnancy. This is a temporary discomfort that will resolve after a few weeks.

Tip: Realize this is normal and try not to put much pressure on your breasts until the tenderness dissipates over the next few weeks. Adjust your bra size if needed. Get a comfortable bra with good support.

- *Frequent urination.* Having to urinate more frequently is common in early and late pregnancy. Your changing hormone levels cause the smooth muscles of the uterus and bladder to relax, increasing the sensation of the need to urinate. In addition, your body is beginning to get rid of waste for two people.

Tip: Plan for more frequent trips to the bathroom, especially when you're involved in activities such as a long car trip, a meeting, or going to a movie. *Do not wait to go to the bathroom.* Holding off will only cause you mental and physical stress. If you experience a burning sensation or pain of any kind when you urinate, or feel that the need to go is urgent but you produce little urine, you may have a *bladder infection.* Report these symptoms to your doctor or midwife.

- *Increased vaginal discharge.* This is caused by the change in hormone levels and is your body's way of making sure the entrance to the uterus is clear of any bacteria.

- *"Morning sickness."* This is the most talked about discomfort of early pregnancy. It is actually a misnomer since it can occur at any time of the day. Many women describe it as feeling like the beginnings of a stomach flu. You feel nauseous—as if you're going to throw up. You may also be actually vomiting at times. Some researchers believe this symptom of early pregnancy is caused by the rapid change in the level of hormones. Other researchers believe it's caused by the way your body breaks down and utilizes carbohydrates. You can't really do anything about the hormones—they're needed to maintain the pregnancy. But you can provide your body with a more constant supply of carbohydrates.

Many women with morning sickness experience it upon waking perhaps because their bodies have been without carbohydrates during an 8 to 10 hour period of sleep. The answer to the problem, whenever it occurs, may be to give the body more carbohydrates. Unfortunately, the last thing you'll want to do when you feel like this is to eat.

Here are some tips for dealing with morning sickness:

1. Make sure you get something light to eat just before bedtime. Graham crackers and a small glass of milk or a few crackers with cheese and half of a banana will prevent your stomach from getting completely empty during the night and will help keep your blood sugar stable.
2. Throughout the day, try to notice when you have the most intense symptoms of "morning sickness," then, in the following days, try to eat something prior to this time period even if you're not hungry. Remind yourself that there may be unpleasant consequences if you don't follow the schedule.
3. Try eating six small meals a day instead of the usual three, or include nutritious snacks in your daily eating.
4. Avoid fried or greasy foods. They may exacerbate morning sickness and they aren't good for a pregnancy diet anyway. Spicy food may also not be tolerated well in early pregnancy.
5. Always carry some crackers, protein bars, or dry cereal with you. You should keep snacks in the car, at work, and in your purse. When you start to feel queasy, eat these carbohydrates slowly and try to get some fresh air.
6. If you feel nauseous, put a cold cloth on your face and take slow, deep breaths to calm yourself. Realize that the anxiety of knowing you may be getting "sick to your stomach" may make the problem worse.

7. Some women learn how to use acupressure. This Chinese method of applying pressure to various points in the body may be helpful in alleviating your pregnancy nausea.
8. Others say that eating foods containing ginger or drinking ginger tea or ginger ale decreases their morning sickness.

If you feel that your morning sickness is unbearable, or if you're vomiting more than once per day, let your doctor or midwife know. Other symptoms to report include producing only small amounts of dark urine, feeling light-headed, and a rapid heartbeat. These may be signs of dehydration. Your OB provider may provide nausea medication to alleviate your distress. A severe case of morning sickness is called *hyperemesis gravidarum*. If you find you cannot tolerate any solid food and most liquids, you will need to be closely monitored by your OB provider.

TRY THIS

Have the following items in your car and at work to help with morning sickness:

- Crackers, dry cereal, and dried fruit in small plastic bags or containers
- A large plastic bag—if you need to get sick while in the car
- Some moist wipes to refresh you
- A bottle of water

Along with the common symptoms of morning sickness, you may experience less common symptoms: unusual food cravings or spotting.

Unusual Food Cravings. You may not have problems with morning sickness but crave unhealthy foods, nonfood items, or may have no appetite during this first trimester. These responses to early pregnancy are all normal.

Tip: If you find you're wanting to eat excessive amounts of foods high in fat or sugar, choose healthy eating menus or meal plans that describe specific meals to prepare and eat. Enroll your husband and family members in the same plan to avoid having fattening food around. Give yourself a tiny reward once in a while.

While some cravings are normal, wanting to eat things such as clay, dirt, chalk, or starch, is called *"pica craving"* and may be caused by a lack of certain minerals and vitamins in your body. Tell your doctor or midwife about any pica cravings. Some women crave ice in early pregnancy. This is not necessarily harmful but may be a sign of anemia and should also be reported to your obstetrical provider.

If you have little or no appetite in the first trimester, try to eat small portions frequently during the day, ignoring your lack of hunger. Learn which foods contain the nutrients your baby needs, and plan to include them in your diet. You may want to make a schedule that establishes when you'll have regular snacks. Healthy snack foods include yogurt, pretzels, trail mix, nut butters, fruit, and raw vegetables.

Spotting. You may notice a little spotting—a tiny amount of red or brownish blood—during the first trimester. Sometimes spotting happens because tiny blood vessels on the cervix break after sex. Spotting can also be caused by a minor vaginal infection. Or it may occur when the fertilized egg implants in the uterus. Most of the causes of spotting are nothing to worry about, but it's important to report all incidences to your doctor/midwife. She or he will determine if any action is necessary.

If you have spotting accompanied by pain in the pelvic area, back, or shoulder, report these symptoms immediately to your OB provider. He or she will want to see you to be sure you're not having an *ectopic pregnancy*.

With ectopic pregnancy, a fertilized egg does not descend into the uterus for implantation. Instead it remains in the fallopian tube and starts to develop there. If the embryo is allowed to remain there, it will rupture the fallopian tube. Once this problem is diagnosed, the treatment is usually successful. If you're diagnosed with an ectopic pregnancy, for the sake of your health, your pregnancy cannot be allowed to continue. Prompt action on the part of your OB provider will ensure that you're able to try and become pregnant again as soon as you desire.

KEY THINGS TO REMEMBER

Symptoms of an ectopic pregnancy usually include:

- Severe pelvic pain
- Severe back pain
- Severe shoulder pain
- Irregular spotting or bleeding.

If you have any of these symptoms, contact your OB provider.

Your Baby's First Trimester

So far we've focused on what's happening to you in this early stage of pregnancy. But what is happening to your baby in the first trimester?

In the first week, a fertilized egg changes into an embryo. This embryo develops a sac that will become the placenta. Once the placenta starts forming, the cells of the embryo begin to differentiate into cells specific to different parts of the human body. Your baby's major organs—the heart, lungs, stomach, and brain—begin to develop. By Week six the major structures of the brain, head, and backbone have formed and the heart starts to beat. Next, the face, eyes, chest, and abdomen are discernible and the bones are no longer soft.

By Week 12 your baby is called a fetus. Brain and muscles are responsive to each other. Your baby will have every major part of its body by the end of this trimester, including its ovaries or testicles. Your baby will be about two and a half inches long and weigh about five-eighths of an ounce. However, it does not look like a real baby yet. It needs the next two trimesters to fully develop and function properly:

- The baby's heart begins to beat, although it's very hard to hear even with specialized equipment.
- The baby's sex can sometimes be determined by ultrasound, but this can only be verified by collecting a sample of amniotic fluid and looking at the chromosomes. If you wish to know the sex of your baby, you'll usually have to wait until the second trimester.
- A major organ is developing in your uterus—the *placenta*, an

organ unique to pregnancy. Its purpose is to provide nutrients to your baby via large blood vessels. The baby's large blood vessels lie next to your blood vessels. Nutrients and oxygen pass through walls of your blood vessels into the placental blood vessels. Your baby's blood does not directly mix with yours. Waste is also transferred from your baby to your system via the umbilical cord that connects your baby's belly button to the placenta.

Important To Do's in the First Trimester

There are seven actions to accomplish during this trimester. In fact, these actions remain important throughout the nine months you will be pregnant. If there are beneficial changes you didn't make before pregnancy, now is the time to make them happen. Every positive action helps you and your baby to a healthier and more enjoyable pregnancy experience. Remember, you're in training for a very physical event, in fact, three physical events: the growth and development of your unborn baby, the birth of your baby, and the care of your body after delivery. If you follow these guidelines, you'll have a much better chance of getting through all of these events with ease.

1. Get early prenatal care with a qualified medical provider/ practitioner.
2. Eat healthy foods. As we discussed earlier, what goes into your body has a major impact on your baby's growth and development.
3. Take prenatal vitamins prescribed by your OB provider. These provide a range of vitamins and minerals, and supplement your intake of iron, calcium, and folic acid.
4. Stay away from harmful substances such as alcohol, tobacco, and illicit drugs, or substances not prescribed by your health care provider.

Tip: If you find it hard to give up an occasional drink with friends or after work to relax, try imagining you're offering the drink to your baby. Ask for a soft drink or fruit juice instead.

5. Get plenty of exercise. Most women don't get enough. Now is the time, when you're "off to a new start," to change your habits. Exer-

cise is often put off by women because they keep thinking they will have more time later to get around to it. Even if you have no idea how you're going to fit one more thing into your busy schedule, sign up for a yoga or a swim class for pregnancy at your local community center. Sometimes the act of enrolling gets you going.

6. Rest. We all know the benefits of rest. We just don't follow through on what we know. Now is the time to go to bed earlier and take naps.

7. Develop a positive attitude at the beginning of this pregnancy and enjoy the journey. Your pregnancy journey may take some unexpected turns, but you don't have to be thrown or discouraged. Continue to keep your OB provider informed about what is happening to you. Trust that you can talk to him or her about any fear or worry, and that your doctor or midwife will help you to get through this journey safely. Everyone's goal is a healthy baby.

Some Special Notes

If you have a chronic illness such as diabetes, talk with your doctor about the impact of the pregnancy on your illness and about your illness's impact on the pregnancy. Make sure you understand what you need to do to stay healthy during the pregnancy. And be sure you know what symptoms to report to your doctor.

If you're 35 or older, or if there's a family history of certain diseases, ask your doctor about genetic testing. Most pregnant women, regardless of age or family history, get a blood test called the *maternal serum alpha-fetoprotein test* (MSAFP). It looks for signs of neural tube defects and Down syndrome. Other tests screen for other genetic diseases (see Chapter 1).

The first trimester passes quickly for many women. As we noted earlier, you may not know you're pregnant during the first six weeks and you may not be terribly bothered by morning sickness or fatigue in the second half. You usually aren't "showing" in the first trimester, and many people may not know you're pregnant. Even if you do have bouts of nausea or feel very tired, your coworkers, friends, and family may not notice that you've changed.

Your Second Trimester

The second trimester of pregnancy runs from Weeks 14 to 27. Many people consider this the fourth, fifth, and sixth months of pregnancy.

Body Changes

This is usually considered the "peaceful time" of your pregnancy. Your morning sickness has probably gone away and you feel you have more energy than during the first trimester. But however "peaceful" it may seem, your body is undergoing more changes:

- You start to "show," meaning your abdomen begins to expand and your uterus pushes forward. You have a pregnant profile.
- You may notice a few "stretch marks" on you breasts, hips, and abdomen. Most of these fade after you have the baby.
- As your uterus enlarges, the two ligaments attached to your uterine muscle need to stretch as if they were rubber bands. Unfortunately, the ligaments do not stretch as easily as the uterus. Any sudden movement you make, even a sneeze, can result in a spasm of pain—a condition called *"round ligament pain."* The ligament's ability to stretch does improve with time. There are several things you can do to alleviate this discomfort. Try to move a little slower when you have a spasm. If this doesn't help, lie down on the side that's painful and massage the area to get the ligament to relax. Round ligament pain usually only happens when you're moving, not when you're in a relaxed position. If the pain does not get better with rest and massage or does not go away fairly quickly, call your OB provider to report your symptoms.
- There will be noticeable changes to your breasts. They continue to enlarge, the nipples and the skin surrounding the nipple get darker, and some women may notice a small amount of clear discharge from their nipples. This discharge is *colostrum*, a highly nutritious fluid that is usually released from the breasts when breast-feeding begins. Having colostrum release before birth is common at the end of the second or third trimester and perfectly normal. Tell your OB provider if you notice any blood coming

from your nipples. It may simply be caused by irritation to the nipple but should be checked out.

- You may notice your cheeks getting rosy, or you may get brownish patches on your face. This is called *chloasma*, or the "mask of pregnancy." You have rosier cheeks because you have more blood circulating. The brownish patches on your face are due to the increase in pregnancy hormones and will usually go away after delivery.
- You may be surprised at the amount of weight you gain this trimester. You'll need maternity clothes. Consider investing in comfortable and quality maternity clothes that you can wear to work. To save money, don't hesitate to ask sisters or friends who are near your size if you can borrow theirs, if they are not in use. You should also commit to purchasing comfortable quality underwear during pregnancy; they will make your physical changes more bearable. If you plan to purchase nursing bras, wait until the last trimester, when your bra size stabilizes.

Tests

You usually have your first ultrasound in the second trimester. (Some physicians choose to do a sonogram in the first trimester.) Midwives may not include a sonogram in their prenatal care. You may request one.

There are two ways to have an ultrasound. The more common is with an *abdominal transducer*. With this method, you must drink several large glasses of water before getting on the examining table, and you refrain from using the bathroom until the procedure is complete, since a full bladder helps get a better picture of the uterus. Once on the examining table, a warm liquid gel is put on your abdomen. A wand or sticklike device called a *transducer* is rolled across the gel and sends sound waves into the abdomen. The transducer transmits a picture of your organs or the baby to a TV screen. Ultrasound does not hurt, but it can be a bit uncomfortable because of the fullness of your bladder.

Another way to do an ultrasound is to use a *vaginal transducer*. This method is helpful for early diagnosis of suspected problems, such as an abnormal placement of the placenta. It also can determine if the length of the cervix might cause difficulties in pregnancy. For an ultrasound with a vaginal transducer, you also will lie on your back on an examining table, but your legs will be in stirrups, as if for a vaginal exam. The vaginal transducer is similar to the size and shape of a tampon. It feels like a speculum used during a pap smear.

Either kind of ultrasound helps your OB provider measure the length of the fetus and confirm how far along you are in your pregnancy. Sometimes after seeing and measuring the baby with ultrasound, your OB provider may change the date your baby is due by a few days. If you're unsure when your last menstrual period started, an ultrasound can help the doctor/midwife determine when the baby is likely to be born. The ultrasound may also help confirm whether you're carrying more than one baby.

Another recommended test is the maternal serum alpha-fetoprotein (MSAFP), also called a Triple screen, which identifies women who should consider further testing for genetic disorders in their babies. A blood sample for MSAFP is usually drawn at a prenatal appointment in the beginning of the second trimester. If results of the MSAFP indicate potential problems, a genetic test, amniocentesis, can be scheduled for the twentieth week of pregnancy. For amniocentesis, a small sample of amniotic fluid is withdrawn and evaluated using ultrasound. Another option for women who need this information earlier is chorionic villus sampling, which can be done as early as 10 weeks. It is usually offered to women who have had a previous child with genetic disorders.

What You Can Expect

The most exciting thing that happens during this trimester is that you'll begin to feel your baby move. The movement will be subtle at first. Some describe it as feeling as though butterfly wings are brushing the inside of the belly. As the baby grows larger and stronger, its movements will become more obvious. Feeling flutters, pokes, and jabs will confirm that you are indeed carrying another human being.

Note the date you first feel your baby move and what it's like. This is a turning point in your pregnancy. It will be a sensation you'll probably never forget, but it's worth putting your thoughts down on paper. Let your doctor or midwife know about it. Later in pregnancy they'll ask you to keep track of how often your baby moves, but for now it's just exciting to feel this other being moving inside you.

Another exciting moment is the first time your partner also feels the baby move, which he might not be able to feel for a few days or even a week after you do. At this stage of your pregnancy, your baby can make significant movements, like flipping over, having hiccups, and even sucking its thumb. Usually your baby's activity will be recognizable to both you and your partner by the end of the second trimester. Feeling the baby move amazes everyone.

Aches and Pains

You may have little discomfort in the second trimester, but a few things could very well begin to bother you.

Occasional *leg cramps* might well occur, due to a change in the way your body uses calcium while you're pregnant. These cramps can be eased by gently flexing the foot while putting weight on it. A heating pad may also help. (See "Exercises During the Second and Third Trimesters," following.)

Veins in your legs may become more visible. These are varicose veins. The increased weight of the uterus during pregnancy causes blood to return from the legs more slowly, swelling the veins. If you indeed notice that your leg veins are more pronounced, avoid wearing tight clothing, and put your feet up as often as possible. Do not cross your legs while sitting in a chair. And when standing in one place for any length of time, move, at least slightly, by shifting your weight from foot to foot.

Increased *nasal congestion* is another discomfort of pregnancy. It's caused, once again, by your changing hormones increasing blood in the veins of your nose. If you have frequent nosebleeds, tell your OB provider. Otherwise, it's probably safe to keep drinking lots of water and blowing your nose gently.

Finally, your partner, while wildly excited about becoming a parent, may find your ballooning figure a reason to decrease intimacy. He may be fearful of harming the baby. You may or may not be interested in having sex, but if you want more physical intimacy, it's important to let your partner know this. You can encourage him to express his changed feelings. Hopefully, whatever the situation is, you can both make adjustments and eventually laugh about the changes you're both going through.

Exercises During the Second and Third Trimesters

Upper Body Stretches (for Strength and Flexibility)

1. While sitting cross-legged on the floor, raise your arms out to the sides to shoulder height and then straight overhead. With palms facing each other. Stretch upward while breathing out. Bring arms down and repeat 5 to 10 times.
2. While sitting cross-legged, raise your arms out to the sides to shoulder height. With palms facing forward, stretch your arms back as if trying to put the backs of your hands together behind your back. Repeat 5 to 10 times.
3. While sitting cross-legged, with arms and hands relaxed, lift your shoulders closer to your ears and gently let them down. Repeat 5 to 10 times.

Pelvic Floor (Kegels) Exercises (Toning Muscles Used for Childbirth)

1. This exercise can be done in any position. The goal is to tighten your pelvic muscles for a few seconds and then release them. To understand what muscles you're tightening, try stopping the flow of urine the next time you go to the bathroom: Those are pelvic muscles you're using around your vaginal area but do not include your buttocks. Do three or four of these "pelvic floor" tightening exercises several times a day.
2. Lie on your back with your knees up and feet on the floor. Place your hands on your navel and hold. Gently tip your pelvis so the small of your back touches the floor. Hold for a few seconds and release. Repeat 5 to 10 times.

Abdominal Exercises

1. Lie on your back with your knees up and feet on the floor. Place your hands on your navel and hold. Raise your head and shoulders off the floor and exhale. Lower your shoulders and head back to the floor. Repeat 5 to 10 times.
2. Lie on your back with your knees up and feet on the floor. Place your hands on your navel and hold. Raise one shoulder and your head as you reach forward with the arm on the same side as the

lifted shoulder. (You're reaching across your body to the opposite knee.) Repeat 5 to 10 times. Repeat this exercise with the opposite shoulder and hand.

Leg Stretches (Leg Cramp Prevention)

1. Lie on your back with your knees up and your feet on the floor. Gently tilt your pelvis so that the small of your back touches the floor. Lift and straighten one leg until it's perpendicular to the floor. Gently point and flex the foot of the extended leg. Repeat 5 to 10 times. Repeat this exercise with the other leg.

2. Stand facing and holding onto a wall. Keeping your hips in line with your shoulders, slide one foot back out as far as possible without lifting the heel off the floor. You'll need to bend the opposite knee and lean forward. Hold for a few seconds. Repeat with the other leg.

Lifting and Posture Exercises
(for Posture and Movement Habits)

1. Always squat or kneel on one leg to retrieve an object near or on the ground. *Never* lean over to pick something up. Bring the object close to you before standing. Use your leg muscles to rise.

2. Stand straight with shoulders relaxed and knees unlocked. It's okay to tighten your abdominal muscles. Walk with your feet parallel to each other.

Back Exercises

1. For your lower back: Sit in a straight-backed chair. Slowly lean forward over your pregnant abdomen, letting your head drop and your arms hang down from your shoulders. Hold for a few breaths and then slowly rise, one vertebra at a time stacking on top of the previous one, until you're upright again and your head is up looking forward. Repeat five times. Do not do this exercise if you feel any pressure or pain in your abdomen or back.

2. For your sides and upper back: Sit cross-legged with your right hand on your thigh above your left knee and your left hand on the floor. Gently pull on your thigh to twist around toward your left side and look behind you. You should feel a stretch on your

side. Repeat five times and then do the same on the right with your left hand on your right thigh.

3. For the whole back and hips: Get on your hands and knees with your weight evenly distributed. With your back straight, gently rock your hips back toward your legs as if you were going to sit on them, hold for a few breaths, then rock forward again. When back in the starting position, curl your back upward like a cat as your head hangs down. Return to a flat back and rock back toward your feet again. Repeat these two movements five times.

Your Baby in the Second Trimester

By the Week 16 your baby's facial features have developed, although the eyes remain closed. It can swallow amniotic fluid and pass urine out of the bladder. Your baby is moving, though you may not be able to detect any movement until Week 20, and its hair is growing, teeth are developing, and the baby may suck its thumb.

At this point in the pregnancy, your baby is about half as long as it will be at full term, or about 10 inches. By Week 24 your baby is thought to be able to hear your voice, music, and other sounds. It can cough and hiccup, and you may be able to tell when these actions are happening. Its body is covered with a white substance called *vernix*, which protects the skin from drying out. There is almost no body fat.

Important To Do's in the Second Trimester

1. Take the time to notice how you are feeling. You're probably feeling pretty good. Write about how you feel and what you hope for the future. With your partner, make a special effort to take time to enjoy being "just the two of you" before the baby comes. If you have other children, engage in some activities or short trips with them, and engage in other activities with your partner alone. You may find it refreshing to spend some personal time away from work, family, and friends before the two of you become "three." Often we're so busy in our lives that we forget to enjoy living.

A special note: If you're not particularly happy during this trimester, if you're crying more or having trouble sleeping, you may be exhibiting the symptoms of depression. Everyone experiences the blues occasionally, but a prolonged period—over two weeks—can have an effect on your pregnancy, and some believe may even directly affect your baby. It's important to seek a diagnosis and get help if it's needed. Let your provider know what you're experiencing.

2. Sign up for childbirth preparation classes. Some kinds of childbirth prep classes recommend getting started in the second trimester. Take your classes very seriously and get your money's worth by practicing with your partner every chance you get. You may believe you don't need classes if you're planning to have pain medication, like an epidural, during labor. But these classes are not only about labor. They'll teach you strategies to get through the last part of pregnancy, prepare you for labor and delivery, and educate you about the postpartum period, including breast-feeding and newborn baby care.

3. See your dentist to complete any work you need or for a checkup. If you've put off dental work, you may experience problems in the later stages of pregnancy since your body demands more calcium during pregnancy, which reduces the amount available for your teeth. And, because of changing hormone levels, your gums can become more sensitive and bleed when brushed. Make sure your dentist knows you're pregnant and when your baby is due. He or she may not want to do a lot of work on your teeth except for routine cleaning. Dentists often prefer not to give any medications or take X-rays during the latter stages of pregnancy. Most dental work is fine during the first and second trimesters, but to be safe, discuss any work to be done with your OB provider.

4. Once again we suggest that you take a pregnancy exercise class, to prepare you for the physical work of labor and to decrease stress. Exercise should be a priority. If you haven't found time to exercise on your own, sign up for and attend a class with other pregnant women. Being with others who feel similarly awkward

or ungainly may help you enjoy it more. You can do the exercises in this book at home, but we strongly recommend that you take a class, such as yoga or water aerobics, outside your home to ensure that you exercise regularly and safely. Finally, ask your husband or partner to gently encourage you to follow up on getting regular exercise.

5. Because you'll most likely feel more energy and strength in this trimester, you may want to finish major projects at work or in your home. This may be the best time to paint the baby's room, for instance, interview for a pediatrician, or find day care or babysitters. If you're planning to move to a new place before the baby is born, you should try to make the move now. Later, in the third trimester, you'll be too exhausted and have too many other things on your mind. Finding and moving to a new place is very stressful at any time. It takes a lot of physical and emotional energy. If possible, you may seriously want to delay this effort until after the baby is born.

6. Watch for any signs or symptoms of preterm labor. Again, because you usually feel so good during this trimester, you might do too much. You may even become exhausted, which is a strain on your body. Preterm labor can occur when you're not taking time to rest and take in adequate fluids. (We'll discuss the symptoms of preterm labor in the next chapter.) Always talk with your doctor about any changes in your pregnancy.

TRY THIS

Make a List of Things to Do Before Your Third Trimester

At about Week 22, list the decisions you need to make prior to childbirth. The list should include:

- The hospital or birthing center where you'll deliver. Write the name and phone number down. Take a tour of the delivery site.
- Sign up for childbirth preparation classes.
- Select your labor coach.
- Decide, if you have a boy, whether you want him to be circumcised.
- Decide if you'll breast- or bottle-feed your baby.

Your Third Trimester

The third or last trimester is from Week 27 to Week 40, or the seventh, eighth, and ninth months. This is the final phase of the pregnancy before the birth of your baby. In this stage, you'll experience many physical demands on your body. Every activity may seem to require a lot of effort.

Aches and Pains

- You'll probably feel as though you can't get enough air in your lungs. This shortness of breath is due to the fact that your uterus is large enough to begin pushing up on your diaphragm—the flat muscle that lies beneath your lungs and abdomen—and the pressure on your diaphragm prevents your lungs from completely filling up with air. You'll have enough air for you and your baby, but until your baby moves down into your pelvis in preparation for delivery, you may feel uncomfortable when trying to take deep breaths.

- You may experience frequent heartburn. In fact, "heartburn," a burning pain in your chest area, is a misnomer because it does not involve the heart at all. In late pregnancy, digestive juices from the stomach may escape into the esophagus because pregnancy hormones have relaxed the smooth muscle around the valve at the top of the stomach that normally holds these juices down. Eating snacks or dividing your eating into more frequent, smaller meals will keep food in your stomach constantly. The food should absorb the digestive liquids and keep them from bubbling up. Heartburn is usually not a serious condition and should go away after the birth of your baby. Your health care provider may have some other suggestions if your heartburn is getting worse instead of better.

- Another problem you may encounter is constipation. Pregnancy hormones have caused the muscles involved in digestion to relax, and as a result, they can't move food through your system as effectively as before. Also, your growing baby is reducing the space for your intestines. And finally, your body is demanding more fluids. All of these factors affect normal elimination and can result in constipation.

Tip: To prevent constipation, drink more water, continue with light exercise, and eat foods high in fiber such as raw vegetables. You may want to try eating two servings of bran cereal a day. Talk to your doctor or midwife if these strategies don't help.

- You may gain the most weight during this part of your pregnancy. About one pound a week is normal. Some of your maternity clothes may no longer fit, and your shoes may feel too tight.

- Each trimester takes a lot of work, but this one takes the most effort. You'll definitely feel the physical demands of this pregnancy—as if you're carrying 20 to 30 pounds of luggage around with you everywhere you go for three months. You are likely to tire more easily and more often, and need more time to do routine tasks.

- You may experience backache from carrying the extra weight of your pregnancy, most of which is in front. It's also because of the loosening of your ligaments. General pregnancy backache can be eased by doing pregnancy exercises and stretches, yoga or water aerobics, heat, massage, and by resting more frequently. Try to do the back exercises described in the second trimester section of this chapter.

- You may have episodes of sciatica, which occurs when the weight of your pregnancy presses on nerves lying close to the spinal column. The nerves become swollen and cause pain in the buttocks and down the legs. Sciatica pain is eased by back-strengthening exercises, alternating applications of heat and cold packs, and sometimes with pain medication. Your OB provider may refer you to a physical therapist.

- You may find it difficult to sleep because you can't find a comfortable position, particularly if, when not pregnant, you usually sleep on your front or back. By the third trimester, your large belly will make it impossible to sleep on your front, and sleeping on your back is not recommended since this position may restrict blood flow to your uterus. Try lying on either side, with a pillow placed between your knees or try placing a small pillow under one hip to tilt your uterus to one side.

- Your blood pressure may rise, causing your feet and ankles to swell. Your face may also look puffy. Continue to have your blood pressure monitored during prenatal visits to ensure that you're not developing pregnancy-induced hypertension. PIH occurs more often in women who have had hypertension before pregnancy or who have a family tendency toward hypertension, but it can occur without these factors. If your doctor or midwife is concerned that you may be developing PIH (see Chapter 11), he or she will give you precise directions about how you can monitor your blood pressure and when to report symptoms.

- You may feel clumsy, and simple tasks may seem impossible. Just bending over to tie your shoes or to shave your legs will be more difficult with a large belly. Ask your partner for help with these tasks.

- As you approach the end of this last trimester, your lungs will have more room because your baby will drop deeper into the pelvis. Unfortunately, this preparation for birth puts greater pressure on your bladder. In other words, your shortness of breath will improve at the expense of your bladder. You'll find yourself having to go to the bathroom often, even during the night. Remember, if you have any pain when urinating, a persistent lower backache, or a strong need to go to the bathroom but only a slight amount of urine, you may have a bladder infection. Report these symptoms to your doctor or midwife.

- You'll feel more frequent and stronger movement from the baby for most of this trimester. In the last few weeks, your baby will be approximately 6 to 7 pounds and 18 to 21 inches long. Your baby now has very little room to move around. But though his or her movements tend to decrease, it's important that you feel the baby moving every day. Your doctor or midwife will be able to tell you the amount of movement you should expect.

- You may begin to feel a few contractions. Occasional contractions are normal in the last trimester. Your uterus is flexing in preparation for labor. If these flexing sensations, the contractions, become more frequent and regular and you are in the earlier part of the third trimester, they could be a sign of preterm labor. Let your doctor or midwife know about them. In fact, it's always a good idea to speak with your doctor or midwife about any new sensations. (We'll discuss preterm labor and what to do about it in Chapter 5.)

Your Baby in the Third Trimester

At the beginning of the third trimester, your baby is fully formed. Nevertheless, he or she still cannot easily survive outside the womb. The last organs to develop completely are the lungs, and they will need all of the remaining weeks to be fully functional. While some babies who are born early have only minor health problems, being born early can be dangerous to your baby. Your baby needs this time in the womb to mature and complete the development of its major organs. Having this time will also mean your baby will be better prepared to fight infections.

A great deal of what your baby is doing in this last trimester is growing. It grows from about 12 inches at Week 28 to 20 inches at fullterm, and now begins to fill out, losing wrinkles. In this last trimester it will grow from about two pounds to six or seven pounds, although you might even have an eight, nine, or 10 pounder! After Week 36, your baby will gain about an ounce a day for the time it remains in the womb.

At first your baby may kick and move about a lot. Its eyes are now open. Closer to delivery, the baby's movements will slow down, merely because, as noted above, there isn't a lot of room left to move around. By Week 36 the baby should be head down in the optimal position for delivery. By Week 40 the baby may have long fingernails and long hair. There is little of the white, sticky material called vernix remaining on its skin. Your baby is ready to be born. You're probably more than ready too!

Important To Do's in the Third Trimester

1. Watch for signs of preterm labor before the Week 37.
2. Go to all your prenatal visits, which become weekly.
3. Continue to attend childbirth classes and practice labor pain-relieving techniques.
4. Finalize plans for getting to the hospital, including alternate routes and alternate people who can help get you there.
5. Finalize who will help you after delivery, how long they'll be available, and where they'll stay.
6. Continue to care for yourself by eating right, exercising, and getting rest.

7. Remind friends not to tell you their exciting, but perhaps horrific, labor stories unless you feel the stories are helpful to your thinking about how your delivery will go.
8. Obtain baby supplies, particularly an infant car seat.
9. Enjoy this last stretch of time before your baby arrives.

What Comes Next

While pregnancy can have unexpected bumps, twists, and turns, we believe that if you're prepared for anything, you'll have a better pregnancy experience.

In the next few chapters we'll provide information regarding the conditions for preterm labor and premature birth. Knowing whether you're at risk for preterm labor, and learning the signs and symptoms, will give you more resources to enable you to protect your pregnancy. After all, when you know what might happen, you also know how to take preventive action.

4

Premature Babies:
Who's at Risk?

 Marjory's Journal

Dear Journal,

I was sent to the hospital in preterm labor at 28 weeks. My pregnancy had been fine until that moment. I asked the doctor what happened. He told me that half of the mothers with preterm labor that he sees have no medical reason to go into preterm labor.

In the first three chapters we've discussed becoming pregnant and what that feels like. But if you've talked with your mother, aunts, sisters, and friends about their pregnancies, no doubt you realize that no two are alike. You may even have heard stories that alarmed you or left you feeling anxious about the outcome of your pregnancy. And so, you might want to know more about what could happen, or perhaps you'd rather not know unless something unexpected does happen. Both reactions are normal.

The purpose of this chapter is to help you assess the possible complications that may occur in your pregnancy, which may lead to preterm labor or premature birth. However, it's important to understand that *all pregnant women* are at risk for preterm labor and a premature delivery, even when they do not appear to have risk factors.

That means that even if your pregnancy has gone perfectly to date, you could begin to have preterm labor weeks before your due date. Your doctor or midwife may be able to discover what is causing this change in your pregnancy. When you know it can happen, you can prepare and know what to do to protect your pregnancy. You'll know why and how to take action.

FACTS
- One in 8 pregnancies ends prematurely.[1]
- Fifty percent of all women who give birth prematurely have no risk factors or likelihood for premature delivery.[2]

Unfortunately, there are many unanswered questions about what causes a baby to be born prematurely. To date, scientists have found no single explanation and no one set of factors that explains why women go into early labor. There has also been no definitive explanation as to why preterm labor occurs more frequently each year, although this trend spans the last 20 years.

FACTS
- Currently each year in the United States, about 450,000 births, or nearly 12 percent, are premature.[3]
- The number of premature deliveries in the United States is rising.[4]
- The number of multiple births—twins, triplets, and more—is rising. Babies born as part of a set of multiples are often premature. From 1990 to 1998, the number of women giving birth to triplets or more doubled. Fortunately, due primarily to changes in assisted reproductive technology methods since 1998, the number of higher multiples (triplets or more) has declined. The number of twins, however, continues to increase.[5]

KEY THOUGHT TO REMEMBER
All pregnant women and their partners should educate themselves about preterm labor and premature birth.

You should be concerned about avoiding preterm labor because it can be very harmful to your baby. While there may be some adverse health consequences for you if you develop a complication that leads to preterm labor, the consequences to your baby if he or she is born too early can be severe.

Low birth weight, which is most often caused by premature birth, is the second leading cause of death in infants of all races and the leading cause of death in African-American infants.[6] Fortunately, steady improvements in obstetrical and neonatal care since the turn of the century has meant that more premature babies are surviving. However, a premature baby may be developmentally delayed and require specialized care for some time.

By quickly incorporating cutting-edge treatments into existing neonatal care, medical specialists are able to prevent many long-term problems of prematurity, but many premature babies must be closely monitored during the first two years of life for potential health problems. A small number of premature babies may develop medical problems—such as cerebral palsy and respiratory problems—that may require lifelong care.

Saving preterm babies comes with a high price. In 1999 the average cost of delivery and hospital care of a premature baby was a staggering $57,000.[7] Everyone involved in the care of mothers and babies agrees that keeping your baby in the womb until full term is your best insurance for a healthy baby. Everyone's goal is preventing premature birth.

Risk Factors for Premature Birth

While all women are at risk for preterm labor, you may have risk factors that make preterm labor more likely. Risk factors are those conditions or circumstances that make you more likely to be in danger of pregnancy complications.

Preterm labor risk factors fall under five categories:

- You have a previous medical condition
- You develop a current medical condition
- Your behavior
- Your environment
- Your age and race

The test at the end of this chapter will help you assess your degree of preterm labor risk. The purpose of the test is to alert you to possible complications in your pregnancy, but your physician or midwife is the best person to evaluate your chances for preterm labor. He or she will be able to address any concerns you might have. In order to better understand what the test screens for, we've briefly described many of the conditions that may affect a pregnancy outcome. More detailed explanations for these complications can be found in Chapter 11.

Medical Risks

Your doctor or midwife will rely primarily on medical factors in your personal history to assess the chances of your having complications during your pregnancy. These medical factors are called *preexisting risk factors*. These are events in your medical history that occurred before you became pregnant.

Your Medical History
Previous Premature Birth. You may have delivered a premature baby with a previous pregnancy. This may have come about because you developed a pregnancy complication such as having a pregnancy with fibroids, preterm premature rupture of membranes, placenta previa, pregnancy-induced hypertension, or incompetent cervix. Because any of these complications can return in a current pregnancy and cause problems, they will be described in the section on current medical conditions. Sometimes the cause of the previous preterm delivery is discovered; often it is not. The single most likely indicator for having a preterm delivery is your having had a previous preterm delivery.

Previous Preterm Labor. You may have experienced preterm labor with a previous pregnancy and received effective care that enabled you to carry your baby to full term. If so, you are still at an increased risk—a 30 to 50 percent chance—for another preterm labor episode with the current pregnancy.[8] Fortunately, your previous experience may make you more aware of similar changes in your body during this pregnancy, and thus alert you to the beginnings of preterm labor.

FACT

If you have a history of preterm labor, you're very likely to experience similar symptoms in this pregnancy. Symptoms commonly occur as much as *two weeks earlier* than in the last pregnancy.

GAIL'S STORY

Gail experienced preterm labor during her first pregnancy when she was 35 weeks pregnant. Her doctor advised her to increase her rest and get more fluids, and he began monitoring her pregnancy more closely. She delivered a healthy full-term baby at 37 weeks. In Gail's next pregnancy, she experienced preterm labor at 33 weeks. Because the earlier pregnancy had turned out fine, she did not contact her doctor. Her labor intensified and she delivered her second baby within a week. The baby was required to spend a period of time in the neonatal intensive care nursery to help with his breathing, temperature control, and mastering feeding from breast and bottle.

A Short Time Between Pregnancies. If your current pregnancy follows closely upon a previous pregnancy, you're more likely to experience preterm labor. Less than two years between pregnancies is usually considered short. Doctors speculate that this may occur because the reproductive organs have not had enough time to recover from the previous pregnancy. Certainly, your physical and emotional stress increases because you're caring for a child under two years old while pregnant.

Previous Miscarriages, Cervical Incompetence, Abortions, Surgeries. When a pregnancy ends before the 20th week of gestation, it is called a miscarriage. A miscarriage can occur for a variety of reasons, but if you've had multiple pregnancy losses, your doctor may diagnose the problem as *cervical incompetence*: a weakness in the structure of the opening to the uterus. The cervix, or opening, may be unable to stay closed and contain the fetus. Cervical incompetence may be caused by the congenital structure of the mother's cervix, multiple therapeutic abortions, or previous surgery or trauma to the cervix. Some cases of incompetent cervix occur for unknown reasons.

Previous Intrauterine Growth-Restricted Infant. If you've given birth to an intrauterine growth-restricted infant (IUGR)—a low birth-weight baby that is slower to develop in size and proportion to its gestational age, it is possible to have another IUGR infant. IUGR infants may be born prematurely but not always. This subsequent pregnancy will be monitored for the risk of preterm labor.

If you've had this or one or more of the other medical conditions described above, your pregnancy may be considered at risk. Your OB provider may monitor your condition more closely. He or she may have you increase your visits to the office or clinic.

Genetic predisposition. Some scientists believe that women may have a genetic predisposition for having low birth-weight babies. They think that if you weighed under five pounds when you were born, you're more likely to give birth to a low birth-weight baby.

KEY THOUGHT TO REMEMBER
It's very important that you tell your OB provider of any changes in your body or any unusual symptoms that are concerning you.

Your Current Medical Condition

Multiple Gestation: Twins, Triplets, and More. Preterm labor and birth occur much more often in multiple rather than singleton pregnancies. A multiple pregnancy means you're carrying more than one baby. Because a number of factors complicate a multiple pregnancy, you have a 50 percent or greater chance of delivering prematurely when you carry multiples.[9, 10] Chapter 10 describes how having a pregnancy with multiples may affect you.

Uterine Fibroids. Fibroids are similar to tumors but are not cancerous. They can grow either inside or outside the uterus or both. The fibroids that can cause preterm labor are those inside the uterus with the fetus.

Abdominal Surgery during Pregnancy. You may require surgery during your pregnancy, which is stressful to your body. Furthermore, some of the medications you may be prescribed before and after surgery can cause contractions and lead to preterm labor. Underlying mild infections resulting from the surgery can also cause contractions.

Preterm Premature Rupture of Membranes (PPROM). This means that the amniotic sac, or bag of waters, breaks before your baby is full term, releasing amniotic fluid. This fluid is necessary to support your baby. Sometimes the amniotic sac will merely leak some of the fluid through a small tear or rip. This leaves you and your baby vulnerable to infection.

Placenta Previa. The placenta, sometimes called the "afterbirth," is the mass of tissue that grows inside the uterus and supplies your baby with oxygen and nutrients via the umbilical cord. Normally, it implants above or at the side of the fetus. *Previa* means the placenta is abnormally attached at a lower position in the uterus. When the placenta is attached low in the uterus or lies over the cervix, it may cause bleeding, which must be watched closely and may require an early delivery to preserve you and your baby's health.

Pregnancy-induced Hypertension (PIH). PIH is high blood pressure, or hypertension, during pregnancy. Your body may have difficulty adjusting to the pregnancy. If your blood vessels are not relaxing and enlarging to accommodate the extra blood volume needed for the pregnancy, the blood is forced through undersized blood vessels and your blood pressure increases. High blood pressure is usually defined as 140/90 or greater.

KEY THOUGHT TO REMEMBER
If a mother had pregnancy-induced hypertension, preeclampsia, or eclampsia in a previous pregnancy, she is at risk for these conditions in a following pregnancy.

JANINE'S STORY

Janine stepped onto her bathroom scale. She was 29 weeks pregnant and felt bloated, and her fingers and toes tingled uncomfortably. Her lower back ached. Her bathroom scale said she weighed seven pounds more than she had the previous week. Her doctor asked her to come to the office. Janine's blood pressure was 150/90. Seeing that she had all the symptoms of pregnancy-induced hypertension, her doctor prescribed complete bed rest. He stressed that she should lie on her left side as much as possible and drink more water to promote blood flow to the uterus. Janine was taught how to take her own blood pressure and to recognize signs that it was rising.

After a week of bed rest, Janine went for her prenatal appointment. Although she felt fine, her blood pressure was still very high. She also had a significant amount of protein in her urine, indicating a more serious stage of the condition—preeclampsia. She was admitted to the hospital, and the doctor on duty decided to induce delivery because the baby's heart rate was slowing. At the gestational age of 29 weeks, he weighed only 2 1/2 pounds and was easily pushed out of the uterus.

While Janine recovered fairly quickly from the preeclampsia, baby Eric remained in the neonatal intensive care unit for 10 weeks.

Infections in the Vaginal and Urinary Tract. You've probably experienced one of these infections at some time in your life. A course of antibiotics usually clears up the symptoms and eases the discomfort. During pregnancy, however, these minor irritations can become more serious problems. Vaginal and urinary tract infections can irritate the uterus, cause cramping, and lead to contractions—the start of preterm labor. Bacterial infections can also lead to dehydration, another cause of preterm labor. Frequent urinary tract infections—two or more within a pregnancy—are considered a risk factor for preterm labor.

Anemia. You may develop anemia during your pregnancy for many reasons. The usual cause is an increase in blood volume in the second trimester that is not accompanied by a proportional increase in red blood cells. This is often a temporary condition. During the third trimester, your body will probably make more red blood cells. Anemia sometimes persists into the third trimester and requires supplemental iron.

Diabetes in Pregnancy. This occurs when your body doesn't have enough insulin to process your body's glucose. Without adequate insulin, excess glucose or sugar builds up in your blood and does not provide enough energy to your cells. You may have already had diabetes before your pregnancy or had a family tendency toward diabetes, and developed it during the pregnancy. However, diabetes in pregnancy can occur with no previous family history. For many women who develop it in pregnancy, diabetes remains for the duration of the pregnancy but usually goes away after the birth of the baby.

Poor Weight Gain or Nutritional Status. Being more than 10 pounds underweight before your pregnancy or having trouble gaining weight during pregnancy puts you at increased risk for preterm labor. If you have poor weight gain your baby will probably lack adequate nutrition. Subsequently, your baby's not gaining the appropriate weight predisposes it to a premature birth.

Your Behavior

Smoking. If you smoke, you're more likely to have a premature infant, a miscarriage, or a stillbirth, especially with your second pregnancy. When a mother smokes, the carbon monoxide in cigarette smoke decreases the oxygen in the mother's blood. As a result, there is less oxygen getting to the baby and oxygen is vital to the baby's development. Babies born to women who smoke are generally smaller than babies whose mothers do not smoke, are prone to low birth weight, and thus at risk for premature birth. If you stop smoking during your pregnancy, you significantly improve your baby's health.

Alcohol Consumption. If you drink excessively during pregnancy, you're probably not eating like you should or the alcohol is interfering with your body's ability to absorb nutrients. Thus your baby is at risk for fetal alcohol syndrome (FAS), a physical or mental developmental delay or retardation. The Food and Drug Administration defines "chronic" as six drinks per day. However, developmental delays are also found in the infants of mothers who drink as little as two glasses of alcohol a day and in those who indulge in occasional binges of excess drinking. If you drink during pregnancy, you have an increased risk of spontaneous miscarriage and still birth, or you may have a low birth-weight baby, or a baby with developmental delays.

KEY THOUGHT TO REMEMBER

Many physicians encourage expectant mothers to avoid any alcohol in pregnancy. Some doctors recommend no alcohol when trying to conceive and throughout the first 12 weeks of the pregnancy, but feel an occasional drink later in the pregnancy will not cause harm to the developing baby.

Use of Drugs During Pregnancy. All drugs, whether over the counter, prescription, or illicit, are strongly discouraged during pregnancy unless prescribed by your OB Provider. Even nonprescription vitamins are not recommended because large doses of over-the-counter vitamins have been found to cause birth defects. Before you take vitamins during pregnancy, talk to your doctor about whether they're right for you.

Street drugs can have a range of effects on your developing baby, from slowing brain growth and causing brain damage to addictions that require your baby to go through withdrawal after it's born. Marijuana, heroin, and other street or illegal drugs are known to cause preterm labor, but the drug most dangerous to pregnancy is cocaine, in any form.

Cocaine causes specific reactions in your heart and major blood vessels, which in turn affects the circulatory system of your baby. It can cause the placenta to tear away from the lining of the uterus, which leads to hemorrhaging. This is called a *placenta abruption*. The blood loss prevents your baby from getting enough oxygen and puts both of you in danger.

KEY THOUGHT TO REMEMBER

Tell your doctor or midwife if you are currently using any medications or drugs or have a history of drug abuse. Some medications and treatments prescribed by your doctor can help you cope with the desire to use illicit drugs.

Environmental Risk Factors

Stress. Stress is getting more attention nowadays. We all know that stress is not good for anyone. In general terms, it makes your body work harder. But now, research has found that stress during pregnancy produces increased levels of *catecholamines*, a hormone. Increased catecholamines can initiate contractions and the onset of preterm labor. Scientists are trying to determine if this is a reliable indicator for preterm labor; that is, one that could be used to predict it. Unfortunately, an economical test is not yet available to measure the hormonal changes brought about by stress.

Your stress may come from personal concerns, job issues, lack of support from family or friends, from thinking about national and international events, and from physical realities such as a job at which you spend long hours on your feet. For example, hospital nurses have been found to have a higher than average rate of preterm births than the general population. Becoming pregnant adds to any existing and ongoing stress. You may not even realize how much stress you're under until it affects your pregnancy.

Work-related stress, as noted above, is not uncommon. Your job may expose you to excessive stress either because the work is physically and/or mentally demanding or emotionally draining. Consider that while you're pregnant, in addition to a demanding workload, you are:

- Carrying an additional 10 to 30 pounds of weight
- Drinking fluids constantly
- Going to the bathroom three or four times more often
- Experiencing periodic sleep interruptions
- Experiencing emotional changes

You may find being able to manage these challenges of pregnancy and work very difficult. Unfortunately, taking time off to alleviate work-related stress may cause the additional stress of worrying about the temporary loss of income or whether you'll have a job to return to.

Check with your employer and see if you can temporarily switch to a job that will allow you less time on you feet and breaks to drink more water and go to the bathroom. You may want to explore going part-time or working from home if possible.

TRY THIS

Get your spouse or partner to carry a 20 pound sack of potatoes attached to the front of his body for one or two hours. He should do normal activities, such as getting in and out of bed, going for walks, driving, etc. Have him describe how it feels.

Stress also occurs at home. Women who work at home are also exposed to excessive stress because of physical, mental, or emotionally draining demands. Having children to care for in the home often requires lifting, bending, and stooping, in addition to their emotional demands. Try to prepare ahead by scheduling child care and help with housework, and seeking out emotional stress relievers such as exercise or even counseling.

Environmental Toxins. Paint fumes, chemical leaks, carbon monoxide poisoning, and other toxins can affect your pregnancy. Living at a higher-than-average altitude can also provoke preterm labor.

Preexisting Risk Factors: Medical, Behavioral, Environmental

Preexisting risk factors have been researched well. Having any one of these factors does not mean you'll necessarily deliver a premature baby, simply that you may be watched more closely by your doctor. You can help your doctor protect your pregnancy by being aware of your potential for risk and by knowing the signs of preterm labor. These are explained in the next chapter.

PREEXISTING AND CURRENT PRETERM DELIVERY RISKS SCREENING TEST

If you're pregnant or planning to become pregnant, stop now and fill out the following checklist on your medical history, current medical health, habits, and environment. These questions will help you assess whether you have any risk factors for preterm labor or a premature delivery. Put a check mark next to all the risk factors you feel you may have, and when you're finished, add up the number of check marks.

Previous to this pregnancy:

_____ I have had two or more miscarriages or abortions while being three or more months pregnant.

_____ My biological mother took a medication, or her mother took a medication, called DES.

In a past pregnancy:

_____ I had a baby who was born premature.

_____ I have had early (preterm) labor: cramping, uterine contractions, treatment with medications, or bed rest.

_____ I had incompetent cervix.

_____ I had PPROM (preterm premature rupture of membranes) or my amniotic sac opened prematurely.

_____ I had placenta previa. (The placenta in an abnormal position.)

_____ I had PIH (pregnancy induced hypertension, or high blood pressure).

_____ I had preeclampsia or eclampsia. (High blood pressure that is unresponsive to medication.)

During this pregnancy:

_____ I am carrying more than one baby.

_____ I was told by my doctor that I have one or more very large fibroids inside my uterus.

_____ I was told by my doctor that my cervix (the opening to the uterus) is soft or is starting to shorten or thin out (incompetent cervix).

_____ I was told by my doctor that my cervix is starting to dilate or open up (incompetent cervix).

_____ I was told by my doctor that my amniotic sac (bag of water) is starting to leak or has a hole in it (preterm premature rupture of membranes, PPROM).

_____ I was told by my doctor that the "afterbirth" or the placenta is covering the opening to my womb (placenta previa).

_____ I was told by my doctor I have pregnancy induced hypertension (PIH).

_____ I have had two or more vaginal infections in this pregnancy.

_____ I have had two or more kidney infections, bladder infections, or urinary tract infections.

_____ I am anemic.

_____ I have maternal or gestational diabetes.

During this pregnancy, two or more of the following are true for me:

_____ I gave birth less than two years ago.

_____ I have had three or more abortions or miscarriages in the first two months of pregnancy.

_____ I am 17 or younger or I'm over 35 years old.

_____ I'm 10 pounds underweight for my height or I was 10 pounds underweight at the start of this pregnancy.

_____ I stand more than 30 percent of the time in my work or I do heavy lifting.

_____ I climb two flights of stairs more than four times per day.

_____ I take care of a child under two years of age most of the day.

_____ I feel I'm going through a lot of stress in my life at this time.

_____ In the past, I have smoked one to three packs of cigarettes a day, or I smoke about this amount ____ (number of cigarettes/day) now.

_____ On average, I drink more than one alcoholic drink per week.

_____ I've had a lot to drink (an alcohol binge) at any point during this pregnancy.

_____ I now use, or within the past five years have used, street drugs (including marijuana, cocaine, heroin, speed, LSD, etc.).

_____ I have not had prenatal care until now or I'm not currently receiving prenatal care.

Congratulations! You've just screened yourself for preexisting or current risk factors for preterm labor and premature birth. If you have any of these risk factors, your pregnancy can still go very well, but, regardless, you should discuss this information with your OB provider.

On the other hand, if, after taking this test, you believe you do not have any preexisting risk factors, you may avoid many of the complications caused by these risks. However, keep in mind that many women who deliver a premature baby have no pre-existing risk factors. Our hope is that, knowing you *may* experience preterm labor, you will prepare yourself for that possibility. Don't despair—prepare! Know the signs and symptoms of preterm labor, which we'll examine in Chapter 5. As you'll see, *early detection* of preterm labor is critical to preventing a premature birth.

5

Signs and Symptoms
of Preterm Labor

 Stacy's Journal

> *Dear Journal,*
> *When I was pregnant for the first time, I remember being worried about all the usual things, like was the baby going to be all right and would labor be really awful. I never thought the baby might come early. During my second pregnancy, that's all I worried about.*

You play a critical role in helping your doctor or midwife to identify early symptoms of preterm labor so he or she can take action to prevent a premature birth. Being able to recognize the symptoms and alert your OB provider will have a positive and beneficial impact on your pregnancy and on the health of your baby.

Many women often know something is wrong or different in their pregnancy. Sometimes they just don't feel "right," even though they're not in pain or uncomfortable. They only know something has changed. When you know about preterm labor, you're more likely to

---

KEY THOUGHTS TO REMEMBER

Remind yourself of the subtle signs and symptoms of preterm labor and of the importance of taking action if these symptoms occur. Knowing about preterm labor will empower you to protect your pregnancy.

identify what's normal for you and what may be an early symptom of preterm labor so your OB provider can take preventive measures to help you in your pregnancy.

Here are the signs and symptoms. You can have one or more of them at a time:

1. *Uterine contractions*. These may or may not hurt. They may feel like a tightening sensation in the uterus. Often this is described as the baby "balling up." The uterus feels hard to the touch, with the firmness of a basketball.

2. *Cramping, like menstrual cramps* before a period. The cramping is often felt in the lower abdomen and may increase in frequency and intensity.

3. *Lower backache*—usually below the waist. It often feels like pressure or aching in the back and comes and goes in a pattern. Over time, it can also feel painful as it moves to the front of the abdomen.

4. *Gaslike pain in the abdomen*, with or without diarrhea. This feels like a stomach flu. This symptom usually shows up in the second trimester.

5. *Leaking water or a gush of water from the vagina*, referred to as ruptured membranes. This wetness can be a constant wetness on the underpants or one big gush of water that runs down the legs.

6. *Bleeding or spotting* on the underwear or when wiping after going to the toilet.

7. *Pelvic pressure*—a sudden heavy feeling in the area between the tops of the legs. This is often described as feeling as if the baby's head has dropped down very low and is putting pressure on one's vaginal area. It is an achy, uncomfortable feeling.

Recognizing the Symptoms

Recognizing the symptoms of preterm labor can be difficult because **they're often quite subtle and mild and can be easily dismissed as the common discomforts of pregnancy.** If you have never been pregnant before, you may be unsure about what a contraction feels like.

You may feel something different but may think it's just one more sensation to get used to as a normal part of pregnancy. Contractions are a normal part of pregnancy when they occur at the right time in your pregnancy (full term) and in the right amount.

Occasional contractions happen throughout pregnancy for all women. So how is one to tell whether these physical sensations are normal or the beginning of preterm labor? Recognizing the symptoms of preterm labor can be a challenge, *but it is the key to protecting your pregnancy, your baby, and yourself.*

When uterine contractions continue for some time, your cervix may begin to change in preparation for birth. When these changes to the cervix reach a certain point, stopping the progress toward an early delivery is very difficult and can lead to the premature birth of your baby. If you're aware of what symptoms to watch for, you're more likely to recognize them and can contact your doctor to be evaluated sooner.

Remember other subtle symptoms such as cramping, gas pains, and backache may also be signs of preterm labor. These may gradually increase in severity or frequency. But even though they become more pronounced or come more often, they may still not be recognized as something to call your doctor about. It's natural to think that these symptoms are not important to report to your OB provider, when they're not uncomfortable or when you think they are something else like a stomach ache from eating something that didn't agree with you. But reporting of symptoms allows your doctor or midwife to determine whether they warrant closer inspection.

Contractions

Labor—both pre- and full-term—occurs when the uterus, which is essentially a very large muscle that contains the baby, begins to contract *or tighten up*. You cannot control the tightening and relaxing of the uterine muscle in the same way you can control the muscles in your hand or arm.

The uterus contracts before full term for several reasons: in response to hormonal changes in your body, with stretching or pulling inside the uterus caused by large movement from the baby, with significant

TRY THIS

Flex your right arm so the muscles on the upper arm tighten and get hard. With your left hand, feel this firmness.

This is how your uterine muscle feels when you're having a contraction.

Sometimes you feel hardness on only one side of your abdomen. This is probably not a contraction but the baby's head or bottom. *A contraction makes the uterus feel hard all over like a basketball, not just in one place.*

changes in your activity, *and for unknown reasons.* Contractions of the uterus can occur at irregular intervals or they can occur in a regular pattern. Whether or not there is a pattern, these tightening sensations are still contractions. This is how the uterus practices for the true labor. Your uterus is a muscle that has to be in top shape to contract enough to push the baby and placenta out of your body.

During full-term labor, the uterus contracts repeatedly to push the baby against the cervix, which is the opening or baby's exit route. This pushing against the cervix helps to dilate, or open, the cervix. When it's fully open the baby can be born. Labor contractions continue after the baby is born, until the placenta is expelled.

Recognizing Contractions

You may be unaware that early contractions are happening. This will be especially true if you've never had a baby before or didn't feel contractions with your last pregnancy. Here's how you can learn about your contractions:

1. If you have an opportunity during a prenatal visit, ask your OB provider to help you feel for a contraction or ask to be placed on a fetal monitor or nonstress test (NST) machine. This machine records contractions you may or may not notice. Ask your doctor or nurse to tell you when a contraction is occurring or is showing up on the fetal monitor. Try to notice any sensations you're feeling during those times.

2. Palpate for contractions. Feeling for contractions is called *palpating*. Contractions usually have some kind of rhythm. First your uterus feels firm, then soft, then firm again, and sometimes you'll feel them form a regular pattern. A contraction may last about 30 to 45 seconds, and if allowed to continue, will progress to lasting 60 to 90 seconds. Sometimes the tightening sensation extends to the upper legs and lower back. Some women describe their contractions as feeling like the baby "balling up."

TRY THIS
Depending on how far along you are in your pregnancy, you may be able to feel a contraction. To feel or palpate for contractions, place both hands on the sides of your abdomen and feel for any tightening or firm "balling up" of the uterine muscle.

3. Be willing to call your provider. The key to avoiding a premature birth is to notify your health care provider as soon as possible if you're experiencing any sign or symptom of preterm labor, or any new sensation that worries you. Call if:

- Cramping, tightening, or contractions occur as often as four or more per hour—regardless of how mild they feel
- Cramping or persistent gas pain does not seem to go away after one hour of rest and after drinking extra fluids
- You have any bleeding, constant leaking of fluid, or a gush of water from the vagina

Early action on your part will assist your doctor or midwife.

What Is Preterm Labor?

If you have more than three weeks to go before your due date and the uterus begins active, regular contractions that appear to dilate or open the cervix, this is considered preterm labor.

KEY THOUGHTS TO REMEMBER

Contractions that can lead to preterm labor are usually those that oc-cur four or more times in one hour and persist even after you drink 16 to 32 ounces of fluid and lie down for one hour. Most doctors and midwives are more concerned when you have six or more contrac-tions in an hour but they know that studies show that women feel only a percentage of the contractions they are actually having. OB providers want to err on the side of caution, so don't discount any kind of contraction.

False Labor

"True labor" occurs when a woman's uterus contracts until the cervix opens and the baby is born. "False labor," often referred to as *Braxton-Hicks contractions*, is labor with sporadic contractions that eventually stop. Telling the difference between the two can be very difficult because the contractions feel the same. One way for you to self-diagnose is to change positions when you feel contractions or tightening. False labor contractions will usually go away after a change in position, such as from sitting down to standing up, or vice versa. True labor is unresponsive to any changes in position.

In preterm labor prevention, "a contraction is a contraction." You may be having "false labor," but these irregular contractions can still

KEY THOUGHTS TO REMEMBER

Once you reach three weeks before your due date, or 37 weeks gesta-tion, you do not need to worry about preventing contractions. At this time you are considered full-term and can have your baby at any time. But before this time, pay attention to the contractions you have.

If you're having more than three contractions per hour, make sure they go away within the next hour or report them to your doctor, mid-wife, or nurse practitioner. Discuss these instructions with your OB provider and follow his or her specific directions.

cause your cervix to dilate if they persist over time. The terms "false labor" and Braxton-Hicks contractions imply that these contractions are nothing to worry about. Not so. Any kind of contraction can be the start of a preterm labor episode. Don't discount them.

The Cervix and Preterm Labor

The cervix is the door to the uterus or womb. Contractions work to open and thin the sides of the cervix so the baby can pass through in delivery. If you're experiencing persistent contractions, your doctor or midwife will examine your cervix for changes. Because looking for cervical change is part of the medical management of preterm labor, we'll describe cervix change in the next chapter. We will address here the matter of having contractions with no cervical change.

You can have contractions that do not cause the cervix to change. These are called preterm contractions, which are different from preterm labor. If you're having contractions but your cervix remains closed after more than one exam, your OB provider may tell you to call only if you start to have more than the usual benchmark of four contractions per hour. For instance, a woman who's carrying twins can have four to six contractions an hour with no cervical changes over a period of two to three weeks. She may be told she can wait to call the doctor until her contractions become even more frequent—perhaps seven or eight contractions per hour. Keep in mind your OB provider needs to make this decision because he or she knows what your body is doing and what your risks are. Don't make the decision to discount contractions because you feel you're having preterm contractions and not preterm labor.

Your OB provider will also want to determine if your higher number of contractions is caused by some irritation to the cervix, such as an infection or semen from intercourse.

If you think you're having preterm contractions:

1. Remind yourself that contractions are normal.
2. Try to determine if what you feel is really a contraction. Palpate or feel your abdomen with your hands to see if it's tightening all over. What you feel may just be baby movement.

3. Try to determine how many contractions you're having in one hour. If you're having one or two an hour, write down the time and duration of each contraction and go about your day, but notice any increase in the number or intensity of your contractions. Let your doctor know about these contractions at your next appointment.

4. Review "Signs and Symptoms of Preterm Labor," above, to see if you have any other signs of preterm labor. Get instruction from your OB provider if you do have other symptoms accompanied with contractions.

5. If you're having four or more contractions an hour, *and you have approval from your doctor*, you should try the self-treatment measures for signs and symptoms of preterm labor below. If this is the first time this has happened, or if your OB provider wants to be notified whenever this occurs, call him or her immediately.

Self-Treatment Measures

Note: *The following instructions are not meant to replace the instructions of your doctor, midwife, or nurse practitioner. You need to get approval before treating yourself.*

Self-treatment is something you can do to try to get your contractions to stop or decrease when they are caused by something minor like dehydration or too much activity. However, as noted in the above warning, talk to your doctor about self-treatment measures *before you need to use them.*

When you notice that you're having four or more contractions in one hour, cramping, backache, or pelvic pressure, try the following self-treatments:

- Immediately drink 16 ounces of water or diluted juice.
- Go to the bathroom and empty your bladder.
- Lie down on a couch or bed on your left side with your feet up for one hour sipping another 16 ounces of fluid.
- Time the contractions and write it down so you can report the amounts, times, and duration to the doctor, nurse, midwife, or clinic.

If you're still having contractions after one hour or you feel a back-ache or menstrual-like cramping, call your doctor immediately. Also, if you have bleeding, spotting, or leaking fluid, you need to call your OB provider right away. Even if the contractions stop and you are feeling better, you need to get more rest and fluids for the remainder of the day.

How Does Self-Treatment Help?

Often, drinking water and lying down will be sufficient to calm an irritable uterus and stop the contractions. You may have gotten busy and forgotten to drink enough fluids. You may be dehydrated, which can cause your uterus to begin contracting. It's very important that you continue to drink at least 64 ounces (eight 8-ounce glasses) of water or other fluids each day. It's also important to take frequent rests during pregnancy. Take time out to put your feet up and just relax. Have a glass of water and a "lie down" a couple of times a day.

KEY THOUGHTS TO REMEMBER

Don't ignore contractions, especially if they seem more frequent than normal. Tell your doctor or midwife about them and ask whether you should continue to follow self-treatment steps when symptoms occur.

Reporting Your Symptoms. Start by telling your OB provider your name, when your baby is due, if you've had any problems in this pregnancy so far, any medication you're taking, and if your cervix had started to change at a previous office visit.

Then report the following:

- All your symptoms (backache, contractions, cramping, leaking fluid, bleeding or spotting, etc.)
- The *frequency* of contractions
- How long the contractions last (duration)
- Whether you've tried self-treatment measures
- How active your baby is usually, and if the activity level is different at this time.

Depending on your symptoms, your OB provider may decide to have you come into the office or the hospital to be evaluated or give you other instructions to follow. However, *if the contractions continue or return, monitor your contractions and contact your OB provider again.* Write down his instructions to remember them.

Erring on the Side of Caution

Claire stood in her half-empty living room watching two movers come down the stairs with her dresser. It was a June day and the sweat dripped down the men's faces and formed dark streaks at the necklines of their T-shirts. Claire rocked from foot to foot. She wished she could be of some help during the move. She was six months pregnant and was not supposed to lift anything heavy. Earlier, she'd made several trips to the car, carrying some lighter boxes. She stopped when she felt the baby do a somersault. At least she thought it was a somersault. She hadn't felt that particular sensation before. There it was again. What was it? She tried to describe to herself the sensation so that she could describe it to her midwife. It felt as if her stomach was rock hard and the baby was balling up, or curling up into a ball, maybe making a flip or a quarter turn. She couldn't decide.

Claire continued to feel the "somersaults" and the "balling up" throughout the day. She decided she must have a very acrobatic baby, and she tried to ignore the queasy sensation that accompanied the baby's movement. She did not realize that the sensations she was having were *uterine contractions*.

Claire and her husband John met the movers at their new home and the unloading began. She couldn't remember which box contained her pregnancy books and brochures, and she didn't think it was necessary to call her midwife to report the sensations. By evening, she and John were exhausted. John noticed that Claire seemed unusually uncomfortable and that she kept rubbing her stomach. He asked if they should call the midwife.

"I thought it was just the baby moving but now I feel like I'm having *cramps!*" she exclaimed.

John called the after-hours number, and when the midwife called back, she instructed them to go to the hospital. They didn't say much to each other on the way to the hospital. Each was afraid of making the other more frightened.

To be continued in the next chapter . . .

You Can Protect Your Pregnancy

It's common for expectant mothers to deny that they're having a problem because they aren't physically uncomfortable or because they fear being perceived as too anxious. Claire, the expectant mother in the above story, did not know what was going on with her body, but she did recognize that what she thought were somersaults were a new sensation. As time went on, she realized that the sensation was not going away and was occurring more often. Her need to protect her pregnancy overcame her need to deny the symptoms, and she sought help.

To give away the ending: As you'll discover in the next chapter, Claire and John were able to avoid a premature delivery. This was because they sought help in time. While their story had a happy conclusion, it would have been helpful for this couple to have known the signs and symptoms of preterm labor.

As expectant parents, you can play a significant role in preventing the premature birth of your baby. There are a variety of medical treatments for preterm labor, depending upon the condition of baby and mother. The next chapter will describe hospitalization and possible medical interventions to stop preterm labor and avoid a premature birth. In most cases, the success of these treatments is influenced by the early detection of preterm labor.

Here are some simple ways to try to avoid preterm labor:

1. Learn the signs and symptoms of preterm labor.
2. Be sensitive to changes in your body that may be signs or symptoms of preterm labor.
3. Notify your OB provider as soon as possible. When they know about possible preterm labor events, they can take measures to prevent a premature birth.

4. Drink at least 64 ounces (eight cups) of water per day to prevent dehydration.
5. Ask your partner to watch for any changes in your comfort level, that you are getting enough fluids, and whether you're stressed or overdoing things.
6. Begin to palpate or feel for contractions as early as 20 weeks into the pregnancy. (Your partner can also palpate.)
7. If you experience four or more contractions an hour, call your doctor or midwife unless directed to do something else.

KEY THOUGHTS TO REMEMBER
Don't blame yourself for episodes of preterm labor. You cannot control your uterine muscle, and preterm labor can occur even when you follow all the recommendations for avoiding them.

You can protect your pregnancy by learning the signs and symptoms of preterm labor. Call your health care providers if you have any questions. There is no such thing as a silly question. Your health care provider wants to know what is happening to your pregnancy.

Episodes of Preterm Labor

Yes, as the title of this final section in the chapter implies, you can have more than one episode of preterm labor. In fact, if you've had an episode of preterm labor or preterm contractions, you are more likely to have more before you deliver your baby. You'll be more prepared the second time around. You'll know how your body feels when having contractions, know the signs and symptoms of preterm labor, and you may know what usually causes and relieves these contractions and other symptoms.

We recommend keeping a record of your pregnancy. If your pregnancy has several episodes of preterm labor, you can keep a contraction log, a list of any medications you're taking to stop contractions, what your doctor has told you about your cervical changes, and the dates of any hospitalizations. You can help yourself through this some-times frightening and trying time by focusing on your goal—getting your baby as close as possible to full term, or 37 weeks.

If at any time you feel you need to be seen or your symptoms are frightening you, call your OB provider and insist on being seen. Your gut instincts are usually very reliable.

6

Preterm Labor: When the Journey Isn't Smooth Sailing

 Susan's Journal

> *Dear Journal,*
> *I made it to 37 weeks — Paul and I will celebrate tonight. Two trips to the hospital and frequent doctor visits were trying but paid off. I'm glad we didn't give up!*

If you report any of the preterm labor symptoms described in the previous chapter, your doctor or midwife may wish to see you in the office or send you to the hospital. Then he or she may:

- Ask you to describe your symptoms, when they started, and how long they've gone on
- Evaluate your contractions
- Evaluate how your baby is reacting to them by monitoring your baby's heart rate with a fetal monitor
- Check your cervix for any changes
- If need be, check for ruptured membranes

Monitoring Contractions and Your Baby's Response

To monitor your contractions, you'll get on an exam table or into a labor chair and the nurse will strap two wide elastic bands or belts with sensors around your midsection. This is a nonstress test, or fetal monitoring machine.

CLAIRE AND JOHN'S STORY (CONTINUED)

Claire was taken to a hospital room and had an IV put in her arm. Two belts were wrapped around her abdomen. The nurse was explaining to Claire that one of the belts was to check the baby's heart rate and the other would determine if she was having contractions.

A few minutes later, Dr. Bell entered the room. He explained that Claire was having preterm labor contractions and said he was glad they'd come to the hospital when they did. His goal was to stop these contractions before they opened up the cervix and delivered the baby.

"What do you mean?" John said. "She can't have this baby—she's only six months along! Will our baby be okay?"

"Your baby will probably be fine, but it's best to try and avoid an early delivery," Dr. Bell replied. He explained that the first thing was to get the contractions to stop.

He examined Claire and found that the cervix had begun to soften. He thought that the extra fluid would be enough stop the contractions.

Three hours later, after the contractions had slowed to two an hour, Claire and John were on their way home. Neither one had the energy to talk. Their new house seemed especially strange and cold. They crawled into bed and tried to sleep.

The next morning, a nurse called to say that the doctor wanted to see Claire again in two days. The nurse reviewed the "Signs and Symptoms of Preterm Labor" for Claire and emphasized that she should drink at least eight ounces of fluid an hour, preferably water, and the importance of rest.

One sensor measures the baby's heart rate and response to uterine contractions. The other measures your uterine contractions—their quality, strength, frequency, and duration. Contractions, if they progress into labor, usually get stronger, longer, and closer together.

Having a lot of very mild contractions is usually referred to as having "an irritable uterus." Data from the nonstress-test (NST) machine will help your OB provider determine whether you are indeed moving into preterm labor, and the likelihood that your body will benefit from intravenous therapy and medications to stop the contractions.

Examining for Cervical Changes

Your doctor or midwife will perform an internal examination of your cervix to see if it has begun changing. The cervix is measured for length, thickness, and dilatation. He or she can *feel* your cervix by inserting two fingers of a gloved hand into your vagina. Some doctors *view* the dilation of the cervix using a *speculum*, the device used to open the vaginal walls during a pap smear. Neither method of examination is painful, but they can be a little uncomfortable. A vaginal sonogram, similar to an abdominal sonogram, is another way to evaluate the cervix. For this, a tampon-shaped probe is inserted into the vagina. Using sound waves, it transmits an image to a monitor resembling a television.

Persistent contractions usually cause the cervix to soften, shorten, and open up. These changes are also called *effacement* and *dilatation*. If your cervix has begun to change significantly, especially in dilating (or opening up), it will not close back up again. Progressive dilatation of the cervix caused by persistent contractions will eventually result in the birth of your baby.

The goal in preterm labor management is to keep the uterus calm—with few contractions, so irreversible changes to the cervix do not occur.

The cervical conditions include:

Softening Cervix. If you put your finger on the tip of your nose, you can feel hardness and a tiny space between the cartilage sections of your nose. This is how your cervix should feel to your doctor or midwife—firm and yet movable. A softening cervix means this firmness goes away. For most women the cervix is usually six to seven centimeters long. As your pregnancy progresses, your cervix begins to shorten very slowly. Significant shortening doesn't usually occur until the last few weeks of the last trimester, *unless you're experiencing preterm labor*. A measurement of less than 3.0 centimeters is considered significant shortening.

Effacing Cervix. Not only is the cervix usually very long, it's also thick. When the uterus begins to have contractions, the walls of the cervix thin out. This is called effacement. The amount of effacement or thinning is reported in percentages. Usually 20 to 30 percent effacement is considered a minor change, while 50 percent effacement is a clear indication of a cervix preparing for birth. At 100 percent effacement, the cervix is "paper thin" and the birth of the baby is near.

Cervical Os

The size of the opening of the cervix, the os, tells the midwife, doctor, or obstetrical nurse how far along labor is. The size of the opening is measured in centimeters. When the os is 10 centimeters wide, the cervix is completely dilated. This occurs just prior to the birth of the baby.

The cervix has two openings, the external os and the internal os. Normally, the external os opens slowly late in the third trimester. If the external os is opening earlier, preterm labor may be imminent. When the internal os also prematurely starts to open, this is a warning signal of early delivery.

Low Uterine Segment

Development of the low uterine segment means the lower part of the uterus thins, stretches out, and begins to fill the upper third of the vagina. The baby's head—or feet or buttocks, if breech—is preparing to descend into the lower part of the uterus.

When the cervix is one centimeter dilated, or more, and you're more than three weeks from your due date, you are having what's called "preterm cervical change."

All of these changes to the cervix and vaginal area are indicators of your body's preparation for birth. If you're exhibiting these cervical changes, you may be sent to a hospital for further evaluation and treatment.

Other Tests for Preterm Labor

Fetal Fibronectin

A gluelike protein, called cervicovaginal fetal fibronectin (fibronectin for short) connects the amniotic sac to the inner wall of the uterus. When fibronectin is found in vaginal fluid, it's an indicator that preterm delivery is possible. A relatively new test, approved by the FDA, cultures a swab of vaginal fluid to look for fibronectin.

The fetal fibronectin test feels like a pap test and does not hurt. If the test is negative for the protein, the manufacturer feels that your doctor can be 95 percent confident that you're unlikely to deliver within the next two weeks. Currently, this test is very expensive. It would be done only when your doctor is quite sure about the probability of premature birth. Some complications preclude the use of this test, such as a cerclage or ruptured membranes.

Salivary Estriol

Another new test examines a sample of your saliva because higher than normal levels of the hormone *estriol* indicate a risk for preterm labor. The test is thought to be about 68 to 87 percent reliable as a predictor.[1]

Currently, you would have the test if you have a higher than normal number of contractions before 37 weeks gestation without cervical changes. The test helps your OB provider decide if you should get more aggressive preterm labor treatment that includes bed rest and medications, or if you do not need these measures because the test is normal and you will probably not be headed toward preterm labor.

Ruptured Membranes

If there's concern that you may have ruptured membranes or that your amniotic sack is leaking, your doctor will perform two separate tests. The first is a vaginal exam with a sterile speculum in which the doctor looks for evidence of fluid from your cervix. You may be asked to bear down as if for a bowel movement to see if any fluid emerges; this is called "pooling." For the other test, the doctor places litmus paper inside your vagina near your cervix. Paper color changes will indicate that amniotic fluid is in the vagina. Sometimes a fluid sample taken from your cervix is viewed under a microscope to see if there is amniotic fluid present. This is called *ferning*, because amniotic salt crystals look similar to a fern plant.

Testing for Infection

Infections of the uterus, cervix, and urinary tract can lead to a preterm labor event. Culturing samples of blood and urine will reveal if infection is present. The tests usually need a period of time for results, so definitive diagnosis cannot be made for 24 hours or even several days. If there are clear indications of infection, such as fever, you may be put on antibiotics immediately pending the results.

TRY THIS

Get your pregnancy notebook and make a list of questions to talk to your doctor or midwife about at your next prenatal visit. This should include:

- What should you do if you have symptoms of preterm labor?
- Should you call his or her office or the hospital?
- What is your OB provider's approach to treating preterm labor?
- Does he or she use tocolytics? What kinds?
- Does the doctor use an NST machine in the office?
- What hospital would you be sent to if you went into preterm labor?

Home or Hospital?

If your contractions have calmed down significantly and your cervix has not made significant changes, you'll probably be sent home with instructions to remain on some degree of rest. You may also be prescribed a medication intended to suppress contractions. You'll probably be asked to return to the office a few days to a week later for reevaluation of your condition.

If, however, after a thorough evaluation, your doctor or midwife determines your condition needs to be further evaluated or treated, you'll be admitted to a hospital. Continuing to experience regular contractions, having ruptured membranes or vaginal bleeding from your cervix, requires special care.

Tertiary Care Hospitals

Whether you're admitted for preterm labor or for other pregnancy complications, you'll most likely be sent to a hospital equipped to handle high-risk pregnancies and high-risk newborn babies. Tertiary care hospitals are those with the most advanced obstetric and neonatal facilities.

You may continue to be cared for by your doctor, or your care may be turned over to a high-risk OB/GYN doctor called a *perinatologist* or *maternal fetal specialist*. If your care to date has been with a midwife, she will usually turn you over to an OB/GYN familiar with preterm labor complications. If a specialist takes over your care, your current OB doctor or midwife will still be called upon for consultation about your pregnancy up to your hospital admission.

Admission to the Hospital

Your OB provider will send you to the Labor and Delivery Unit of the hospital. The nurse there will usually send you to a screening or intake room and start a hospital chart on you by asking various questions about your current condition and your pregnancy in general. You'll probably have an experience similar to what you had at the doctor's or the midwife's office:

- You'll be asked a number of questions, examined, and asked to provide blood, urine, and vaginal fluid samples.
- You'll have your vital signs taken (blood pressure and temperature), which will tell the doctor if you have signs of infection that may be causing the preterm labor. Signs of infection include a rapid heart rate or an elevated temperature.
- You'll be attached to a monitor that records the fetal heart rate and uterine contractions via a nonstress-test machine.
- The following laboratory tests may be ordered:
  - Complete blood count (CBC): low white cells indicate infection, low iron indicates anemia, low platelets indicate possible high blood pressure and a potential for bleeding
  - Electrolytes, for dehydration, sodium, or potassium imbalance
  - Urinalysis and culture, for elevated protein and glucose levels
  - Vaginal and rectal culture, for Group "B" streptococcus (looks for infection)
  - Cervical culture, looks for Neisseria gonorrhea and chlamydia
  - Wet prep for trichomoniasas, looks for infection

- Hepatitis B or C test, looks for infection
- HIV test, looks for infection
- An intravenous drip will be started in your arm to prevent you from getting dehydrated. It also supplies you with liquid calories to give you and your baby energy and medications without repeated injections. And last but not least, the IV is in place in case an emergency line becomes necessary.
- You'll have a cervical examination. These can be very uncomfortable because the best time for the doctor to examine your cervix is at the peak of a contraction, when the cervix is the most open. If you have placenta previa (placenta at the opening of the cervix), you usually will have ultrasound exams because of the risk of bleeding.
- An ultrasound is usually performed to more accurately gauge the length of the cervix, the amount of amniotic fluid, the location of the placenta, the position of the fetus or fetuses, the condition of the fetus or fetuses, and to estimate its (or their) weight and size.

Treatment for Preterm Labor

The results from your nonstress test and sonogram make up your baby's *biophysical profile (BPP)*. This profile looks at the heart rate, muscle tone, movement, ability, and frequency of breathing movements or chest wall movement, and amount of fluid in the amniotic sac surrounding the baby. The information is translated into points, meaning each measurement has a score on a scale of zero to 10. A healthy BPP is a number between 8 and 10. If the score is below 8, the test is usually repeated at a different time of day. A baby's slow responses could be from his or her taking a nap when the test was performed. The profile is repeated to rule this out.

The BPP tells the doctor how your baby is doing at that moment and also how well developed he or she is at this point. If your baby needs to be delivered early, your doctor will have a good idea of how well your baby will do after birth.

Diagnosis

When all of the samples have been gathered, tests started, and your condition stabilized, you and your partner will meet with your doctor or the specialist assigned to care for you and your unborn baby. You will get an initial explanation of the situation and the doctor's recommendations for treatment.

Who *Are* These Medical People?

Who cares for you in the hospital depends on you and your baby's situation. If either you or your baby is having complications, specific professionals will help evaluate and care for you both. Your doctor or a perinatologist may coordinate your care with the advice of these other specialists.

The long list of specialists includes surgeons, cardiologists (heart), gastroenterologists (digestive tract), infectious disease specialists, and neurologists (brain). For the babies there are pediatric versions of the above, plus neonatologists (specialists in caring for sick newborn babies), audiologists (for hearing), and opthamologists (for vision). To help all of these specialists, there are radiologists and lab technicians, who process the tests and analyze the results along with or for the doctors. And of course there are the nurses, responsible for communicating any changes in your condition to the doctor and for following through with the doctor's instructions for your care. In teaching hospitals there are also medical residents—doctors who are there to learn a medical specialty.

Learning the Lingo, Asking Questions

In the course of your pregnancy you will have learned many new words that describe the changes your body is going through and that describe the development of your baby. The medical terminology may have been hard to understand at times, but the nurses, doctors, and midwives involved usually try hard to ensure that they're being understood.

Occasionally, however, when a woman's condition changes, there may not be enough time for the medical staff to explain what's happening. And in an emergency situation, where time is important or the problem has not been fully diagnosed, the difficult-to-pronounce or hard-to-spell terms used by the doctors and nurses can be scary. In addition, if you have to stay longer than 24 hours in a hospital you'll probably have several different doctors and nurses taking care of you, and each may explain things differently.

In the midst of all this, you and your partner may have to sign consent forms for procedures you may not fully understand. So you might well ask: How can you help with the decision making if you don't understand what's going on?

For starters, don't accept being in the dark about what's going on. Don't be a passive partner in your own and your baby's medical care. Ask your doctor and the nursing staff to give you information in terms you can understand. This is your right as a patient.

The different teams of caregivers should speak with you frequently about your care and make sure you understand what's happening to you. If they don't, ask questions. And if you aren't sure whether you understand something, ask for clarification. Don't wait until you're totally frustrated and beginning to question the care you are receiving. They won't know you don't understand if you don't let them know.

Changing Treatments

You may not respond to the treatment and medication the way your doctors hoped you would. Your plan of care may be modified as a result. You may find that a course of care or a medication your doctor ordered only an hour ago is going to be changed the next hour. These changes can be unsettling for you and your family. You don't know what to pin your hopes on. One minute your doctor is telling you that things are stable, and the next, he or she is saying that the baby may have to be delivered prematurely in a day or two. You might well feel you're on an emotional roller coaster.

A woman's condition while in the hospital can change very rapidly, and thus the treatment and management of preterm labor must progress with the same rapidness. Decisions need to be made with minimal delay. But if you know, in general, what's usually done to avoid a premature birth, and you understand that the decisions are important and may require immediate action, you'll be better prepared for the experience.

Length of Hospital Stay

The medical staff will try to discover what's causing your contractions and will try to stop the threatened preterm birth with fluids, bed rest, and medication. Hospitalization to stop preterm labor may last for only 24 hours—just long enough to stop the labor and to observe you for a length of time. Or it may last several days to several weeks.

Unfortunately, sometimes the cause of preterm labor cannot be discovered, or you might have developed a complication that needs ongoing treatment. Sometimes, preterm labor cannot be arrested without complete bed rest and the help of tocolytics administered and monitored in a hospital. In these cases, hospitalization may last until the end of the pregnancy.

Tocolytics

Many physicians treat preterm labor contractions with a medication group called *tocolytics* (pronounced "to-co-lit-icks"). These are medications used to try to stop preterm labor from progressing by stopping the uterus from contracting. There are many different types of tocolytics, and all act a little differently on your body. However, all of them interact with chemicals in the body, particularly calcium, to relax the uterine muscle. Calcium is needed for muscles to contract. When calcium is blocked or rendered inert, the muscles—particularly the uterine muscle—cannot contract.

There's a great deal of study and debate on the effectiveness of tocolytics. Research has shown that they seem to work best when administered soon after preterm labor symptoms start and for short periods of time. Halting or slowing contractions gains the physician time to administer *glucocorticoids*, also called glucocorticosteroids, or corticosteroids. These steroids are used to speed the development of the baby's lungs and other organs (see "Corticosteroids," following). Tocolytics, are important both in delaying a preterm delivery for as long as possible, allowing the baby more time in the womb, and providing time for these important steroids to take effect.

Who Will Get Tocolytics

Not everyone with preterm labor gets tocolytics. Use of tocolytics depends on your condition, your medical history, the current medical literature that your doctor bases his or her care upon, and what's happening with the baby. However, the following expectant mothers may receive them. Those:

- Between 20 and 36 weeks gestation in their pregnancy
- With at least two contractions in a 15 minute period
- With a cervix dilated less than five centimeters
- With no signs of amniotic fluid infection
- For whom the risk of premature delivery outweighs the risk of prolonging the pregnancy.

Corticosteroids

If preterm delivery seems likely, your doctor's goal is to maintain the pregnancy long enough to give you, by injection, a course of steroids. The medications betamethasone or dexamethasone are glucocorticoids or corticosteroids, commonly known as steroid shots. They cross from your system into your baby's. They work specifically by having the lungs begin producing surfactant, allowing the delicate lung tissue better elasticity during breaths.

Getting a single course of steroids means having two or four steroid shots, which must be given at 12 or 24 hour intervals. It's important to try to maintain the pregnancy longer than 24 hours after the last shot, to allow the medication time to be effective.

Having a Full-Term Baby

Even a few days can make a difference in the overall health of a baby. Every effort is made to prolong the fetus's time in the womb to allow for more development of its organs, particularly the lungs. The degree of development of the lungs is the most critical factor in determining the health of a baby born prematurely. A baby's lungs are usually mature enough to function without medical support after 34 weeks gestation.

Immature lungs are susceptible to several diseases, the most prevalent in premature babies being neonatal respiratory distress syndrome, an inability of the lung tissue to expand and contract with breaths.

There are several causes of RDS. Sometimes a premature baby's lungs lack enough functioning tiny air sacs called *alveoli*. Inhaled oxygen crosses through the alveoli into the bloodstream, and carbon dioxide crosses from the bloodstream into the alveoli to be exhaled. If there aren't enough working alveoli, this important process can't occur efficiently.

Another cause of RDS is *hyaline membrane disease*. HMD is a lack of *surfactant*, a fatty or soapy substance produced in the lungs of full-term babies that coats the surface tissue of the lungs and enables them to stretch and contract with breaths.

Monitoring Your Condition

Monitoring your condition and finding the best medication for you is an ongoing process. Your care will include:

- Continually evaluating the baby via a sonogram and nonstress-test machine and updating the resulting biophysical profile.

  As described earlier in this chapter, the NST machine is used for evaluation when you first come to the hospital and frequently thereafter. It records the frequency of your contractions and checks the baby's response to them. Most important, the NST will be used after every treatment, such as the administration of tocolytics, to tell your doctor how you're responding. It will also be used if you feel a change in your body that might signal an increase in contractions or other problems. And finally, when the doctor has given you medication that seems to be effective and feels you're stable and can go home, the NST will be used once more to confirm his or her findings.

- Retaking your vital signs, such as blood pressure, pulse, temperature, and respiration. Not only are these important measurements of how your body is responding to the preterm labor, but

they will tell the doctor how you respond to the tocolytics they
give you.

- Continuing intravenous fluids.
- Continuing (sometimes) frequent cervical examinations to discover if your body is getting ready for delivery. This will most often be done the traditional way, by manual exam.

Discharge from the Hospital

Based on how you're responding to the treatments, your doctor has
three choices about the final outcome. You can be sent home with or
without medication, continue to be treated in the hospital, or deliver
your baby.

Factors that make a difference about whether you can be discharged
from the hospital include:

- How far along you are in your pregnancy
- Having a negative fetal fibronectin test result
- How well the treatments are preventing your cervix from dilating further
- How well you and your baby are doing with the hospital treatments

Assessing and reassessing your condition will continue for as long
as you're in the hospital. If at any point your doctor feels you can go
home, you'll be discharged with explicit instructions for your continuing care during the remainder of your pregnancy. This includes
degrees of activity permitted, amount of bed rest prescribed, medications, fluid, and nutritional requirements.

If your doctor feels you should stay in the hospital, it is because he
or she feels it's the best place to ensure the continuation of the pregnancy and to monitor the condition of the baby. If your doctor recommends delivering your baby, it's because that seems the best option
for preserving your health and that of your baby.

Remember, keeping a baby in the womb for as many days as possible is the ideal. However, in some cases the feeling is that the baby will
be better off being delivered. You and your partner will be included in
this important decision. Your doctor will explain why he or she thinks

delivery is best, how the baby will be delivered, and what complications might occur. Your doctor will also arrange to have a neonatologist—a specialist for preterm newborns—meet with you.

The Neonatologist and NICU

When there's time, you'll meet with the neonatologist, who will explain the health challenges a premature baby faces and what care it will receive in the special newborn nursery. The Neonatal Intensive Care Unit (NICU), often referred to phonetically as the "Nick U," is basically an intensive care ward for newborns. There are many reasons babies go to it, but being born prematurely is a common one.

The neonatologist will describe the specific condition of your baby, what health problems are expected, if any, and what the specialists plan to do for your baby once it's delivered. The neonatologist may suggest that your partner visit the NICU before your baby is delivered.

Your Baby in the NICU

If your baby must be delivered early, both of you will be able to visit him or her in the NICU as often as you like. Visiting the NICU can be very scary the first few times. It's a surprisingly noisy place, with babies attached to monitors that beep often and insistently. It's also surprisingly dark, as this is thought to benefit the babies' vision. You must scrub your hands and arms with disinfecting soap and wear hospital gowns over your clothing before you enter. These measures minimize the spread of germs that would be dangerous to your fragile newborn.

The NICU nurses are very family oriented. They know you and your baby need to bond in the first few days. In addition, it's felt that your baby may get stronger faster and be healthier with your touch, smell, and the sound of your voice. To promote contact between you, the nurses will have you participate in the baby's care, such as feeding, holding, and talking to your baby. Your visits to the NICU will also prepare you for taking care of your baby once it goes home.

TRY THIS

Call the hospital you're planning to deliver at and see if you can take a peek at the NICU. This will help you see the reality of having a baby prematurely. Ask the nurses to point out a baby that is about the same gestation as your baby at the time of your visit.

Preserving Your Baby's Health

Everyone involved in your pregnancy has the same goal: avoiding a preterm delivery in order to give your baby the best possible start in life. Sometimes that means you'll have to endure hospitalization, unpleasant medications, and the stress of being in a rapidly changing situation. Sometimes a premature birth is unavoidable. Fortunately, there are many treatments available to help preterm babies survive and be healthy. By knowing what's likely to happen, you can be a major player in preserving your baby's health.

If you're discharged from the hospital after a preterm labor episode, you should:

- *Drink plenty of water*—16 to 32 ounces per day—unless instructed otherwise by your doctor, to prevent dehydration.
- *Take the time to fully empty your bladder,* to help prevent contractions or a bladder infection.
- *Get plenty of rest throughout the day.* Some physicians will prescribe a degree of bed rest. See the chapter on bed rest for more details.
- *Make sure you understand exactly how and when to take the medication,* if you're discharged with a prescription for tocolytics. You should also know the side effects, if the medication conflicts with any others you take, when to call the doctor, and what to do if you forget to take a dose.
- *Keep your follow-up appointment,* usually two to three days later, or as directed by your doctor.

And be sure to get specific instructions about when to call your doctor regarding the symptoms of preterm labor or the side effects of any medication you've been given.

7

Preparing for Birth—
the Last Leg of Your Journey

 Sonia's Journal

> *Dear Journal,*
>
> *I'm 38 weeks pregnant and feel enormous. The baby feels like she has moved down. At least I don't have as much heartburn anymore. I keep wondering how it will go. Will I be able to do it? Will I scream, curse, or make a fool of myself? Will I know it's starting? How will Brian be? There, I just felt a contraction. It's not bad. I don't mind it. Mom has been babying me these last few days—great meals and little treats of lotions and soaps. It's so nice. She says she'd rather not be in the room for the birth but wants to be nearby. I guess she's a little nervous too. I want it to start and yet I don't want it to. I can't believe that some-time in the next two weeks or so we're going to be meeting our baby girl.*

Think back to the first few weeks you were pregnant. You've changed a great deal and learned a great deal, and now you're facing perhaps the most exciting part of this pregnancy journey—the birth of your baby. You've already made some of the preparations needed to complete this journey. Now it's time to finalize your decisions, since some may need to be communicated to your OB provider. Written or not, these final decisions are part of your birth plan.

Finalizing Your Birth Plan

Your original birth plan was an outline of the way you'd like your pregnancy and delivery to go. As the months went along, you may have gathered more information from friends and other sources and amended your plan. For instance, you may have initially wanted an epidural to alleviate your labor pains during delivery, and now you want to hold off on taking pain medication. Or vice versa.

As you near your due date, make final changes in your wish list. Discuss them with your obstetrician, doula, and/or midwife if these changes will impact on your OB provider's care. You'll feel more relaxed and ready to focus on labor itself if your birth plan is complete. Consider resolving the following items before you begin labor:

1. Do you want a circumcision performed if you're having a boy?
2. Will you breast- or bottle-feed your baby?
3. Who do you want to have present at the birth?
4. How do you want to document the birth?

We'll go into these issues, presenting the pros and cons. You should certainly explore other sources of information. Either before or after you consider the above topics, you can help clarify your considerations by doing the following:

- In your pregnancy journal or a notebook, write down the questions listed above.
- Get your partner to do the same on a separate piece of paper.
- Answer the questions separately in your book or on paper.
- There are no right answers to these questions. They are designed to help you explore and share your feelings about these issues.
- Seek more information on these issues from your doctor or midwife.
- Compare your answers.
- If you don't agree on some answers, try to decide who will be most impacted upon by the issue.
- Try to find common ground.

Do You Want a Circumcision Performed?

Many couples nowadays know before delivery whether they're going to have a girl or a boy. If you know that the baby will be a boy, and if you don't know the sex of the baby, you need to discuss ahead of your arrival at the hospital whether you'd like to have your baby circumcised. If the answer is yes, the minor surgical procedure can be done by a doctor in the hospital. You may prefer to have it performed by a religious leader of your faith. If you're having a birthing center birth, you must make arrangements at a different facility because midwives do not perform circumcisions.

Circumcision is an elective procedure. It is not medically or legally necessary. Most families choose this procedure based on religious or social custom. Muslim and Jewish peoples have a long history of circumcising their males. Families practicing these religions usually plan to have the circumcision performed in a religious ceremony sometime after the baby has been discharged from the hospital or birthing center. The majority of males in the world are not circumcised, but the majority in the United States are, though this social custom has been changing here. More couples in the U.S. are now choosing not to have their sons circumcised, because they know it is not medically necessary.

Will You Breast- or Bottle-Feed?

Organizations concerned with maternal and infant/child health strongly encourage you to breast-feed your baby. The American Academy of Pediatrics' policy statement on breastfeeding recommends that women breastfeed their infants until the infants are twelve months old. It further states that women should be encouraged to continue beyond twelve months if both mother and child want to keep breastfeeding.[1] Breast-feeding is believed to be beneficial to both your baby and you.

Benefits to Your Baby

Breast milk provides complete nutrition for your baby with just the right amount of calories, protein, and vitamins, and it's easier to digest than commercially produced formulas. It provides immunity from diseases, and as a result of breast-feeding, your baby may develop fewer allergies. Most current literature agrees that breast-fed infants are less likely to have ear infections and learning disorders and may possibly have higher intelligence and a reduced risk of acquiring "type two" diabetes later in life. Breast-feeding has psychological benefits as well. It requires more contact between you and your baby, and therefore it establishes or enhances the bond between you.

Benefits to You

Breast-feeding has benefits for you as well. When you breast-feed, you'll need to sit down and hold your baby. This forces you to rest periodically. While you're resting, the hormones released by breast-feeding assist your uterus with closing blood vessels that were exposed in childbirth and in toning the uterine muscle. Breast-feeding also delivers calories to your baby from your body, and losing these calories may help you get back to your pre-pregnancy figure faster.

Choosing to Breast-Feed

Breast-feeding is accepted and encouraged in most societies in the world. An accepting attitude and the expertise of other family members and friends greatly helps a new mother adjust to effective and comfortable breast-feeding techniques. With general approbation, it is of course easier for a new mother to fit breast-feeding into her life.

According to the American Academy of Pediatrics, in 1995, only 59.4 per cent of new mothers were nursing upon leaving the hospital and only 21.6 per cent were still nursing six months later.[2] Why don't more U.S. women choose to breast-feed? There are several possible explanations. To breast-feed successfully you need three things: good role models, accurate advice, and commitment. Considering good role models, for instance, most women do what their mothers and sisters did, and in the United States that often means bottle-feeding.

Why Bottle-Feeding Became Popular

In the early 1960s, drug and commercial food companies developed a milk formula for newborns. The new formula had properties similar to breast milk and replaced a canned milk formula that had caused multiple milk allergies and had no supplemental vitamins critical to the health of a newborn. This new formula supplied good nutrition to infants who did not have a mother or whose mother was unable to breast-feed. It was also advertised as a convenience to mothers who wanted to spend more time with older children or who were working outside of the home.

A lot of women chose this new option—formula feeding—as a way to free them up and still provide a healthy diet for their babies. At the same time, physicians were bombarded with information on bottle-feeding and formula. Soon, many obstetricians knew more about bottle-feeding than breast-feeding and steered their patients toward bottle-feeding.

Pediatricians knew the health benefits of breast-feeding over bottle-feeding but were often not in contact with mothers until the first baby examination, and by then many mothers had already made the decision to bottle-feed. In addition, some pediatricians found themselves recommending bottle-feeding for babies who were having problems with weight gain or for mothers having problems nursing. With bottle-feeding, a doctor could gauge the amount of formula a baby was taking in. In contrast, with a breast-fed infant, the doctor had to estimate the baby's intake by how long the baby nursed and the amount of wet diapers.

Since the 1960s, the medical community has found other ways to assess a baby's intake of breast milk. The pediatrician is most concerned that the baby is gaining weight and does not show signs of dehydration. There's been a great deal more research into the benefits of breast-feeding rather than bottle-feeding an infant. As a result, U.S. obstetricians and pediatricians now recommend breast-feeding over formula feeding.

This is an example of the accurate advice we mentioned above, as one of the three elements that lead to successful breast-feeding. But you may be encouraged to breast-feed by your OB provider yet be surrounded by well-meaning friends and family who don't know how to support your decision. They may not be able to effectively reassure you that you're doing the right thing at three in the morning when your baby doesn't seem to be latching on or your breasts are sore. Or your friends may even become noticeably uncomfortable when they see you nursing your baby in public places. This is where commitment comes in: You may feel you have to defend choosing to breast-feed, and to persist with it in the face of societal barriers.

Commitment and Support

You may experience some of these barriers to breast-feeding your baby:

- Being uncomfortable or embarrassed when you breast-feed in a public area, even if your breast is completely covered.
- Lack of day care at your worksite, which would allow you to continue breast-feeding your baby throughout the day.
- Lack of a private space in the work environment that allows you to use a lactation pump to maintain your milk supply and to store and freeze the breast milk for your baby at a later date.
- Misconceptions or myths about the effect of breast-feeding on your lifestyle or on your body. Two popular myths are that breast-feeding can cause your breasts to sag or will tire you out.

Of course, breast-feeding for you may not be easy, natural, or even comfortable. Sometimes, particularly at first, it can be downright difficult. And you may never get to that imagined bliss that some mothers profess it is. You might feel at times that the only reason you persist is because you've been told it's healthier for you and your baby, and better health may not seem good enough in the face of so much that is discouraging you from continuing.

If you want to breast-feed, don't try to go it alone. Seek help and support from your health care provider, who can also refer you to organizations dedicated to encouraging breast-feeding. Lactation consultants can offer suggestions on explaining the benefits of breast-feeding to friends and family, allay your family's fears about the effect of breast-feeding on your body, and help you solve your working environment/breast-feeding issues. Most important, they're experts at making breast-feeding a rewarding experience for you.

Successful Breast-Feeding Preparation

We strongly recommend you take a breast-feeding class before your baby is born to familiarize yourself with the process. Once your baby is born, you can request that a hospital lactation consultant come to your room to coach you through your first efforts. If you're having a birthing center delivery, your midwife is trained in breast-feeding technique and will offer you immediate coaching.

Another preparation is to ask friends and family for their experience with breast-feeding, even if it was unsuccessful and, especially if it was. They will give you ample warning that it may not be easy. Many women report that they weren't told that they might not fall into nursing "naturally." Faced with initial difficulties, some got discouraged and gave up too easily. Others say that 'breast-feeding preparation" prepared them for the possibility that it might not be a breeze, and so they were more motivated to persevere. Still other women will tell you they didn't worry about preparing and it was a snap anyway. For them, breast-feeding was indeed natural and easy.

Another breast-feeding preparation is to line up someone to talk you through your first sessions after you get home. This person will keep you motivated. One magic phrase or suggestion from her might give you the means to keep on trying a little longer and achieve successful breast-feeding.

With all this preparation, your breast-feeding experience could be the bliss you're hoping for. Ultimately, it's better for you to know that breast-feeding can be a challenge; that with accurate information, a knowledgeable coach, support from your family and partner, and determination, you can be successful. Get support before and after the birth; it's a worthwhile effort. This is a gift only you can give your baby!

Choosing to Bottle-Feed

It's important to understand that it is not wrong to bottle-feed your baby. Bottle-feeding is definitely a good way to give your baby good nutrition.

You may not be able to breast-feed because of an illness, or because medications you take may not be good for your baby. You may try breast-feeding and feel it's just not for you. Or your baby may never get the hang of breast-feeding and may prefer a bottle. For any of these reasons, your baby will need formula, and he or she will flourish.

If you or any of your children were bottle-fed as a baby, you know that giving your baby formula will be fine. Certainly, there are benefits to bottle-feeding. It allows others to feed your baby and may allow you to do other things like rest or spend time with your other children. It means you might be able to sleep at night when the baby cries, because your partner can take care of the feeding. And your partner will get to hold and feed your baby more often, aiding in the establishment of their special parent-child bond.

In fact, someone should always hold your baby while he or she is being bottle-fed. Your baby could choke if it's fed while in the stroller, car seat, or crib. And propping up a bottle for your baby also means you're missing out on valuable cuddling time.

Whom Do You Want with You in Labor?

You probably realize, or your family and friends have told you, how intense and emotional labor is. You can and should be very particular about whom you choose to be in the labor room with you in addition to your partner. Choose someone who will give your partner support by getting him food and drink and stepping in as a coach when he needs a break.

Once you're home, you'll want to focus on caring for your baby and getting your strength back. Ideally, someone who will help you with the care of your other children, cleaning up the house, or preparing meals. Decide if this person can give you positive advice and feedback about caring for your baby and yourself. Choose someone you believe will add positively to this joyful and important time.

How to Document the Birth?

You may want to document this very special time with a video camera, photographs, or voice recordings. But you will need to focus on having your baby, and you'll want your partner's focus to be on helping you. Thus, it may be best to ask another family member or friend to be in charge of documenting this event. You will also have time to take photos after your baby has arrived. Many hospitals offer a newborn baby photo service. Another way to capture memories of this event is to bring a baby-welcoming book for the nurses, doctors, family, and friends to sign.

Vaginal Birth After Cesarean Delivery

There's one more thing some of you will have to decide before your labor and delivery. If you've given birth before, it may have been by cesarean delivery. In many cases, you can try to have vaginal delivery with your current pregnancy. Reasons to want vaginal birth after cesarean delivery, or VBAC, include avoiding the risks of major surgery, having a shorter recovery time, and avoiding the risk of infection, or you may just want to experience a vaginal birth.

You may not be able to attempt VBAC. Your doctor or midwife will look at the medical records of your cesarean delivery to determine if you can. Talk to them about your options and about the risks and benefits.

Labor and Delivery

Okay, the big day is approaching and you are excited and nervous. What can you do about your nervousness?

- *Learn more about what to expect.* This will help you minimize fear of the unknown. Reading and rereading this chapter and other sources of information, and talking with your doctor, nurse practitioner, or midwife, will prepare you for this big event.
- *Take a childbirth preparation class.* You will learn how to use relaxation and distraction to assist you during labor. You need to practice these techniques regularly with your partner.
- *Take an exercise class.* You can continue to help your body prepare for this major physical event by keeping it moving. If you haven't taken any classes during your pregnancy, try an exercise class specifically geared to pregnant women, such as yoga for pregnancy. If activity is restricted by your doctor, check with him about trying the stretches in Chapter 3.
- *Use positive visualization.* Practice imagining the successful birth of your child. Being able to imagine it happening will help you relax and focus during the real event.

Physical and Mental Preparation

Your attitude about labor and delivery is very important. Think of yourself as an athlete getting ready for a race or contest. You want to *condition your body and your mind* for this event.

FACTS

For labor, you will need:

- A positive attitude and commitment to take the time to prepare for this birth.
- A supportive coach. Someone you can talk to, whom you feel comfortable touching you, is not squeamish, has time to practice with you, and will encourage you to prepare and practice.
- A childbirth preparation class.

Childbirth Preparation Classes

A childbirth preparation class will provide you and your partner tools and information to help you manage childbirth. Taking these classes is a good investment of your time and money. These classes will:

- *Prepare you for labor and childbirth.* Most classes include a tour of the hospital or birthing center, and many show a film of the birth of a baby.
- *Reduce your fear of the unknown.* If you know what to expect, much of your nervousness will dissipate.
- *Teach you relaxation techniques* that will help preserve your vital energy and strength, and help decrease the discomfort of contractions.
- *Teach you breathing exercises* to ensure that you and your baby have adequate oxygen during the strenuous work of labor. These exercises will also help you relax.
- Most classes provide training in visualization or imaging.

You may already know you'll be having your baby by cesarean delivery. Because you will still have to go through some parts of labor, childbirth preparation classes are still valuable. You'll learn what will happen leading up to and through your cesarean. These classes will answer your questions about a hospital delivery, how to relax during labor and during the surgery, and about pain management and recovery time after a cesarean. You may want to inquire about childbirth preparation classes specific to having a cesarean.

Visualization or Imaging

An important tool used in labor and delivery is "imaging," or visualization. This is a technique used to help focus your attention toward comfort measures and away from the pain, discomfort, and overwhelming feeling of a loss of control brought on by the contracting uterus during labor.

Visualization was first used in France during World War II, when laboring mothers had to deliver without pain medication because there was a shortage. It has been found to be effective during labor and is also used as a behavior modification technique in the treatment of other medical conditions. It takes concentration and practice to perfect, but many women are surprised at how beneficial it can be during labor.

Many athletes spend a good part of their training time working with visualization, imagining themselves going through an upcoming event. A star basketball player might be told to close his eyes, lie down, and concentrate on visualizing himself in the most important game in his life. He's told to recognize the "fear of failure" that most of us have when we know how important our success is at a particular time. In the player's case, he may fear he's not performing as well as he can, that he'll miss the game-winning shot or foul out. He's told to *see himself shaking off that fear*, getting back into the game, making the key shot, and playing the best game of his career. He is told to recognize how he feels and to see himself as being successful, smiling, hearing everyone congratulating him, and even how the trophy feels in his hands.

The player is told to practice this visualization often, so that when he hears the music start just before the game or hears the basketball hit the floor, he immediately goes into a winning mode.

Visualization in Labor and Delivery

Some "self-help" theorists feel that "if you can see it—you can have it." If you can see yourself getting through a difficult time, then you can convince yourself that you can actually do this in real life. This means keeping a positive attitude and realizing that giving birth is manageable and achievable. On the other hand, if you can't believe you can be successful, you'll convince yourself you won't do well, and consequently, you will struggle during this event. A big part of success is convincing yourself that you can achieve what you want. These theories work for getting successfully through labor.

Try this visualization exercise:

- Visualize yourself realizing that labor has started and that you're becoming anxious about the impending labor and birth process. Then visualize yourself getting control of yourself and telling your partner what's happening. See yourselves working together to contact your doctor and loading up the car.
- As you see yourself at the hospital, you feel anxious again, but then you recognize the room from your hospital tour and begin to feel in control again.
- As the contractions get stronger, you feel your fear increasing, but you begin using your relaxation techniques from childbirth class and you feel stronger again.
- Later, you may see yourself having very strong and regular contractions, feeling a loss of control, having extreme pain during labor, or fearing that the labor will never end. Then you'll see yourself *shaking off the fear* and getting into what you have to do in labor. Your coach is jumping in and helping you get comfortable, giving you ice chips, and talking clearly and calmly to you.
- When the contractions are strong and difficult to deal with, visualize yourself using the breathing techniques to get through the labor pains. You find yourself getting very tired, but you persist.

You hear someone say you are "complete," and you visualize yourself starting to push the baby out. You hear the baby cry, and in a moment, the doctor hands the baby to you. You can't believe your eyes. Your baby is so wonderful. You have completed your journey.

- You need to recognize how this will feel, what your sensations are; you need to see yourself smiling and everyone congratulating you. You have succeeded, and you have your trophy—your newborn baby in your arms. You can smell, see, and touch this wonderful little baby—your baby. You've done it. You are successful.

TRY THIS

Tape record yourself talking your way through the labor and delivery as though you're coaching yourself. (After doing the following exercise, you'll have a better idea of what you want your partner to say or do that will help you. Let him know this and have him carry a list of these suggestions in his wallet.)

- Start by recognizing what you fear.
- Record yourself telling yourself that you can do this, that you can get through labor, and that you will! Say your words with confidence and authority.
- Next, talk to yourself about what you may encounter and how you'll handle it.
- If you start to feel the hard, strong contractions, tell yourself: "Great. These are the most effective contractions and will help me get this baby out. I'm ready for them!"
- Tell yourself: "Now I need to use my breathing to stay in control."
- Congratulate yourself for your success.
- Tell yourself you are almost at the end.
- Tell yourself your baby will be here very soon.
- You can feel the baby's soft little face on you.
- See yourself sitting back after the labor and birth is over. You're tired, but very, very happy.

FRIEDA'S STORY

Frieda was at Week 38 and ready to have her baby. She was thrilled when she found out she was in labor. She'd gone with her husband Jake to the hospital to have a nonstress-test evaluation. Frieda's nurse practitioner was concerned that she hadn't felt the baby kick as he normally did, but by the time they got to the hospital, the baby was kicking away, so there was no need for the test. Frieda noticed, however, that she was having lots of contractions. She was admitted, and the doctor discovered that she was four centimeters dilated. The contractions were uncomfortable, and Frieda began using her visualization training from her childbirth class.

As each contraction came on, she told herself to see and feel the relaxation she'd felt on their recent beach vacation. She remembered the spot because she'd felt calm and happy and relaxed there. She set herself the mental task of rediscovering every detail of the beach at each contraction, and used this self-distraction to get through the painful parts of the birth. Between contractions, she could relax and talk and be present in the room.

This worked out fine until a particularly big, hard contraction came and her water broke. This freaked her out. She was upset about the amount of water, that she was so messy, and that she felt exposed. She was hurting and, worst of all, felt that she'd lost control when she lost her concentration. For a while, she couldn't recreate the feeling of well-being that the beach vacation had given her. But then Jake jumped in and reminded her of the sound of the waves at the beach, the smell of saltwater, and the warmth of the sun. He rubbed her legs to calm her and keep her warm.

Slowly, Frieda got herself back into the routine of relaxing and imaging. At five o'clock she was given an epidural, and she settled back to enjoy the rest of the birth. Soon, the nurse could see the top of the baby's head and summoned the doctor. Before Frieda knew it, she was holding her new baby girl and smiling at Jake. She had successfully used her visualization, relaxation, and breathing techniques learned in childbirth class to help her with the labor and the delivery of her baby.

Pain Relief

As you near the end of your pregnancy, be sure to discuss with your doctor or midwife your options for pain relief during your delivery. Sometimes you and the doctor can predict what you'll need, and sometimes changes during labor will mean that you won't have a choice. It's important to keep an open mind about the pain medications used in labor.

Perhaps you would like to have your baby without any pain medication because you feel that a narcotic-free delivery is better for your baby. You may also feel that having anesthesia will alter the experience of giving birth, or that you won't feel in control of the situation. On the other hand, you may know that you have a low tolerance for pain, and thus believe that you'll feel more in control if you have pain medication. You know yourself best. What will make your birth experience the best for you?

To help you decide about pain medication, it may be useful to know that women have different levels of tolerance for pain during labor. Some experience a great deal more discomfort or pain than others and become stressed and extremely tired. Others can handle pain more easily and thus are less affected by the stressfulness and overwhelming experience of labor.

Research has documented that there are differences in pain tolerance. Having a high tolerance for pain doesn't make us stronger or braver than others. Nor does it mean that those of us with a low tolerance for pain are weaker. Knowing your level of pain tolerance will help you decide about pain medications.

A Birth Plan Without Medication

If you've opted for a midwife delivery in a freestanding birthing center, you should plan to have a delivery without anesthesia. If you're having a doctor-assisted hospital birth, anesthetic medication is an option, but you can request that it be withheld—in which case, make sure your doctor or midwife know you prefer not to use pain medication *before* you go into labor.

To be successful in achieving a goal of giving birth without medication, get plenty of physical and mental preparation by attending your childbirth preparation class and practicing. Some classes offer specific exercises for having a medication-free birth.

You may want to consider hiring a doula (described in Chapter 1) to serve as a coach, advocate, and knowledgeable partner during labor and delivery. A doula has seen labor before and has specific methods that help women in labor, and this alone may reassure you.

If, during the labor and delivery, you remain convinced that you do not want any medications, having made your feelings known to your partner, nurses, midwife, doula, and doctor will help them to support you in your resolve.

KEY THING TO REMEMBER

If at any time you change your mind and want pain medication, you shouldn't feel that you've failed. If you're a first-time mother, the experience of giving birth is something you have not gone through before and therefore you can't really know what you're able to handle. And even when this is a second or later birth for you, the labor may be different from your previous experience. Do what helps you get through labor and gives you a positive experience!

Pain Relief Options

In a hospital setting, most pain medications are available. However, your doctor will know which medications are not an option for you because of your medical history or because of where you are in the labor process. Some medications, if given too soon, can slow down or stop your labor.

In a freestanding birthing center, pain relief options include relaxation and breathing techniques, massage, showers, whirlpool, and sometime analgesics. Anesthetics are not available in birthing centers. Many women choose to give birth with a midwife and are successful in delivering their babies without medication.

Some women choose to use a combination of the above comfort measure along with medications. Talk to your OB provider about your preferences and remember the goal is to have a healthy baby and a positive birth experience.

Analgesic and Anesthetic Medications

You should become familiar with the different kinds of labor medication and how they will affect you and your baby even if you do not plan to use medications. That way, if medications are requested or become necessary, you'll know their purpose and effect.

There are two types of medications used in labor and delivery: *analgesics* and *anesthetics*.

Analgesics, such as Demerol, give you pain relief from the contractions during labor by directly affecting the brain and central nervous system via your blood. They will help you relax between contractions but will not numb any part of your body. They significantly reduce the pain of labor but usually do not take it away completely. Possible side effects include drowsiness and difficulty concentrating. They're not given just before delivery because they may slow the baby's reflexes and breathing. This is an excellent choice for short-term pain relief or if you cannot have anesthesia.

Anesthesia (regional or local) affects only the area of the body where it is given. The laboring mother remains awake for the birth of the baby. Administering any kind of anesthesia requires a physician, and this medication can only be given in a hospital. Possible side effects include headaches, backaches, tachycardia (rapid heart rate), a drop in blood pressure, and cessation of labor. If labor stops or slows, you'll need another medication (Pitocin) to induce labor.

Epidural Block

Epidural anesthesia is the most commonly used pain relief in hospital births. An epidural injection numbs the lower half of the body from just below the waist to just below the knees, but particularly the perineal area. This is the pelvic area from the pubic bone in front to the rectum in back and between the hipbones.

To receive an epidural, a small area of your lower back is washed with antiseptic, and the skin is numbed to prevent your flinching from the needle stick. The anesthesiologist inserts a needle attached to a flexible tube into your lower spine in a space outside your spinal cord while you round your back and exhale. The tube delivers the anesthetic to your lower back after the needle is removed.

An epidural:

- Helps ease the pain of contractions as well as the pain that comes from the baby moving through the birth canal.
- Is also used in larger doses for a cesarean. Having an epidural makes it possible for you to remain awake for the surgery.
- Can slow labor or even stop it because it affects the quality of the contractions. If this occurs, you'll need a medication (Pitocin) to induce labor.
- Will also numb the lower back and legs. You can move your legs once the epidural is inserted and secured in place, but you won't be allowed to walk around.
- Is continuous or occasional pain medication. With the tube in place, continuous small doses or occasional doses can be given without another injection.
- May be given in reduced amounts. You may be able to ask your doctor for a smaller than usual dosage of medication. Having less than the full dosage can give you pain relief and still leave you feeling in control of your progress during labor.
- Allows you to feel only pressure during contractions, not pain.
- Usually doesn't prevent you from pushing the baby out when it is time.
- Is not usually administered in vaginal deliveries until you're dilated four centimeters or more. Starting an epidural sooner may slow down the labor or even stop it altogether.
- May cause your blood pressure and the baby's heart rate to drop. This is usually avoided by providing intravenous fluids and having you lie on your side to improve blood circulation.
- Can cause some soreness in the back after the anesthesia wears off. This soreness will disappear with time.

Spinal Block

Spinal anesthesia is very similar to an epidural but is used mainly for cesarean deliveries or for deliveries that seem likely to need a vacuum or forceps extraction.

A spinal block:

- Numbs more of the body, usually from just below the breast down to the feet.
- Is injected into the lower spine, directly into the spinal fluid, while you're sitting up.
- Is usually administered only once, just before the baby is delivered.
- Will cause a loss of all muscle control, including control of abdominal muscles. It affects your ability to push.
- Lasts several hours.
- Has side effects similar to an epidural.

Pudendal Block

A pudendal block numbs only the "birth canal," or vagina and vulva. It alleviates the discomfort of the delivery, not the labor.

A pudendal block:

- Is administered when the baby is about to enter the birth canal or vagina and be delivered.
- Is injected near the nerves on the sides of your vagina.
- Does not provide any relief from the pain of your contractions.
- Does not interfere with pushing.
- Usually has no direct effect on your baby. The area will remain numb for the stitching of the tear or episiotomy.
- Is considered one of the safest forms of anesthesia.
- Rarely results in serious side effects.

General Anesthesia

General anesthesia is sometimes used for a cesarean birth, but usually for emergency deliveries when the baby needs to be taken out quickly. You may have general anesthesia for a cesarean if you are unable to have spinal or epidural anesthesia. The medication can be given through an IV line or in gas form with a mask, or sometimes both.

General anesthesia is usually not performed "electively." Any kind of surgery that requires anesthesia involves some risk, and so doctors do not use general anesthesia unless it is medically necessary. General anesthesia can affect your baby by slowing its reflexes and breathing and causing sleepiness.

Final Preparations

By the thirty-seventh week of pregnancy you will be armed with a great deal of valuable information, know the value of having a positive attitude, and be physically ready for the birth experience You are ready to pack your *Labor Bag*. It should include:

- Important phone numbers
- Insurance information
- A nightgown that is adaptable to breast-feeding
- Robe
- Slippers
- One or two bras; nursing bras if you plan to nurse
- Toiletries
- Books or magazines, if you like to read
- Three or four pairs of underwear
- Heavy days sanitary pads (the hospital will provide very large pads)
- Eyeglasses/contact lens case
- Baby book
- Birth plan
- Snack for the coach
- A disposable camera with a flash
- Some coins for vending machines or telephone calls

The hospital will provide hospital gowns, sanitary napkins, and some toiletries. It will also provide diapers for the baby. Birthing centers do not usually provide these supplies. Many baby product companies provide a gift pack with disposable diapers, wipes, free formula samples, and other goodies for you in the hospital and hope you'll continue to use their products.

Getting to the Birthing Center or Hospital

It's always a good idea to know alternate routes to your hospital or birthing center. Try driving the most direct route in both rush and nonrush hours. Also, line up someone else in case your partner is not available when you're told to go to the hospital or birthing center.

Preparing for Your Baby's Homecoming

Select the outfit you want your baby to wear home from the hospital and a blanket, but leave them at home so they don't get misplaced or rumpled. Your partner can bring these items when you and the baby are ready to be discharged.

Buy a baby's car seat and have the salespeople at the store or someone in your doctor's office demonstrate how to use it, install it, and remove it from the car. Your hospital or birthing center will not discharge a baby if there is not an infant car carrier in the car. Some hospitals have loaner car seats you can rent until you make your final decision to buy one. This is an important purchase and may require some comparative shopping and research. Try to have this item several weeks before you're due to deliver.

Labor and Delivery Overview

Go back to the idea that you're on a journey through pregnancy. This final leg will take you through some dramatic new terrain. To prepare for this experience, let's review what happens in labor and delivery.

Full-term birth occurs between 37 and 42 weeks of pregnancy. Preparations for delivery, however, have begun well before your baby's birthday. Labor starts sometime in the three to four weeks before you actually have the baby. Your body makes specific preparations that take time, so that the changes are not painful to you or harmful to the baby.

The changes that will eventually lead to the birth of your baby are at first quite gradual. Scientists still don't know for sure what makes labor start, but it's thought that the baby initiates the changes in your body that prepare it for labor and birth, that it's your baby that decides when it will be born. However, your hormones play a significant role in the onset of labor. When the time is right, your hormone levels begin shifting toward those hormones that promote contractions rather than inhibit them. One of the hormones, oxytocin, helps your body make stronger and more effective, regular contractions. Your body also begins to produce prostaglandins, which are key players in softening your cervix for dilation. The increasingly stronger contractions begin to push your baby's head against your cervix and it starts to open up.

Around the thirty-fourth week of pregnancy, most babies move into the head down position. This is called the *vertex* position. Some babies do not get into this position and remain with their bottoms or feet down near the cervix, in the *breech* position. Another, rarer occurrence is when the baby remains lying sideways in the womb in a *transverse* position. See Figure 7-1.

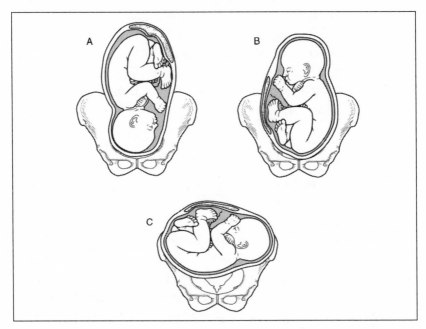

FIGURE 7-1 Diagram of baby positions: (A) vertex, (B) breech, and (C) transverse.

If you've passed the thirty-fourth week of pregnancy and your baby is not vertex or head down, your doctor or midwife can have you do some specific measures or exercises. The "knee chest" exercise in particular has been effective in getting babies to turn to the vertex position before labor begins.

If these exercises are not effective, your doctor can attempt a procedure called *external cephalic version.* To do this, you may have medication to suppress contractions. With ultrasound to guide the doctor and monitor your baby's response, and with the help of another member of the staff, the baby will be manually pushed out of the breech position (feet or buttocks down), into the transverse position, then into the vertex position. You cannot have this procedure if your baby is too big, you're very close to your due date, or if you have other pregnancy complications.

External cephalic version can be uncomfortable, but many women have gone though this procedure without problems. Risks from the procedure include premature labor, premature rupture of membranes, small blood loss for the baby or mother, or fetal distress. But these complications are rare.

If this external cephalic version is not successful and you go into labor with your baby in a breech or transverse position, your doctor has two alternatives. One is to deliver your baby by cesarean delivery. The other is to attempt a vaginal breech delivery. Some babies can be delivered vaginally in a breech position. If your physician is experienced with this type of delivery, if you and your baby are stable, and if it appears that your baby's head and shoulders will not have a problem fitting through your pelvic bones, you can attempt to have a vaginal breech delivery. Because nowadays complications from delivering babies by cesarean section are rare, some doctors will recommend a c-section as the safest way to deliver a breech position baby.

Labor

You have been having mild contractions throughout your pregnancy even if you did not recognize them. As you near the end of your journey, you may begin to feel them more often. At some point, irregular contractions become regular and early labor begins. You may be worried you won't know when you're in labor or won't know what to look for. Most women eventually recognize contractions. The difficulty lies in discovering if your contractions are true or false labor.

In the beginning, contractions are usually mild. You feel as if you're having cramps during your period. They later become more noticeable. They will have a definite beginning and an end. You may have irregular contractions, which last about 20 to 30 seconds and come in an irregular pattern, but usually not closer than about every 30 minutes. These are often called Braxton-Hicks contractions or false labor. In fact, there is nothing *false* about them because they are indeed contractions, even if they do not lead to the delivery of your baby. Braxton-Hicks contractions can be uncomfortable and usually occur when you're tired; at the end of a day, for example. A change in position will often make them go away.

Early true labor contractions come at regular intervals. At first they may occur about 10 to 15 minutes apart. As more time passes, these contractions become stronger, longer, and closer together. Your doctor or midwife will tell you when you should start timing your contractions and when you should call to report them. Some OB providers instruct their patients to start timing contractions when their frequency begins interfering with your ability to concentrate on other activities. Your OB provider will want to know the frequency and duration of your contractions to determine how far along you are in early labor.

Timing Contractions

Timing your contractions is fairly easy, but it works better when you have someone to help you. You'll need a piece of paper, a pen or pencil, and a watch or clock that keeps track of the seconds and minutes, preferably a standard clock with a second hand, rather than a digital clock. To time contractions:

- Note and write the time when the contraction starts. For instance, write 10:01:01 a.m.
- Write when the contraction ends; that is, when you can't feel the discomfort anymore or when your uterus gets soft again. Let's say

the contraction ended at 10:01:16. The contraction from beginning to end lasted 15 seconds. *This is the* length, *or* duration, *of
one contraction.*

To time the frequency of contractions or how often they are
coming:

- Note the start of the first contraction; in our example above,
10:01:01 a.m.
- Note the time when the contraction ended: 10:01:16.
- Now note the time the next contraction starts, 10:16:01, which
is 15 minutes later.

This information tells you that the first contraction lasted 15 seconds and that the contractions are 15 minutes apart. If the contraction that started at 10:16:01 ended at 10:17:01, the second contraction
is one minute long. If the second contraction started at 10:16:01 and
the next started at 10:31:01, the contractions are still 15 minutes apart.
**The frequency of contractions is measured from the beginning of
one contraction to the beginning of the next.** When you call to
report that you think your labor has started, you can say you're having contractions every 15 minutes and that they're lasting one minute.

When You Think You're in Labor

Make sure you understand how soon your doctor or midwife wants you
to call when you think you may have started labor. Most OB practices
tell their patients to call when the contractions are lasting one to two
minutes (duration), are coming every five to ten minutes apart (frequency), and have been going on for over two hours. Some doctors
instruct you to call when you can no longer walk or talk through a
contraction. If you have a family history of fast labors, you've had a
fast labor before, or if you live a considerable distance from your delivery location, you may want to contact your doctor or midwife earlier.

A clear sign of labor is the rupturing of the membranes or the
"breaking the bag of water." This is usually accompanied by more frequent contractions, although you may not have noticed contractions
before the rupture.

Your bag of water can burst suddenly. You will experience this as a gush of clear fluid from your vagina that continues to leak. Or it may break gently and you may just feel a steady trickle of fluid on your underpants. When your bag breaks, your body is usually moving into the next phase of labor. Your OB provider will want you to be under his or her care for this stage and will instruct you to come to the hospital or birthing center.

Call your doctor or midwife's office immediately if you think your bag of water is broken or leaking, or you notice the fluid is dark green or has blood in it. These are indications of conditions that may need immediate medical care and attention.

Other Signs of Labor

By Week 36 you are probably seeing your midwife, nurse practitioner, or doctor every week. Your OB provider is checking that:

- Your baby's position is head down and tucked into your pelvis.
- Your cervix has started to dilate (open up) or efface (thin out).
- You've lost the mucus plug.

You may be asked if you have noticed a small amount of pinkish, brownish, or slightly bloody mucus on your underpants. This is the "mucus plug." Until the later part of the third trimester of pregnancy, thick mucus blocked the opening to your cervix. As your due date approaches, this plug breaks up and passes out of your body. This is usually a very clear sign that your body is preparing to begin labor—perhaps within hours, and usually within days, although it may leave your cervix as much as a month before you actually have your baby.

KEY THINGS TO REMEMBER
Signs of Labor

- Frequent, regular contractions that do not go away with a change in activity and have been going on for over two hours
- Mucuslike vaginal discharge that may have blood or pink tinges in it
- Continually leaking fluid from your vagina

Going to the Hospital or Birthing Center

Depending on the information you provide about your contractions and labor, and your distance from your place of delivery, your OB provider will tell you if it's time to come to the hospital or birthing center.

There are several things you can do if you're told it is too soon to leave for the hospital or birthing center. Ask your OB provider if you can eat a light snack such as crackers and soup and drink fluids with electrolytes, like soda or Gatorade. If you have a doula, alert her that your labor has started and confirm whether you'll meet her at your home or at the hospital. Don't forget to remove any valuable jewelry you're wearing. You may want to try going for a slow, easy walk around your neighborhood. Have your partner go with you. The goal is to get your body relaxed and ready for work. Don't overdo it. You'll want to save your energy for the labor.

If you're given the okay to go to the hospital or birthing center, sit in the car on a large towel in a semireclined position. Do not lie flat during the car ride. The towel will prevent soaking or staining the car seat if your "bag of water" should break on the way or if you're spotting. Don't forget your "Labor Bag."

Arrival at the Hospital

When you arrive at the hospital or birthing center, you'll be met by a nurse or midwife and escorted to a triage room or birthing room and helped out of your street clothes. You will be asked about your contractions and what you've had to eat and drink. Your vital signs will be checked: blood pressure, temperature, and pulse. They will be checked periodically throughout labor and delivery, usually every hour, but more frequently if any are out of the normal range. You may also be asked to give a urine sample. These procedures give your OB team information about how your body is reacting to labor.

Next, your doctor or midwife will perform a physical examination. This will give your OB provider information about your baby's position, whether your pelvis can accommodate the baby's head, the timing and pattern of your contractions, how far your cervix has dilated and effaced, and whether your water has broken. If you're having a doctor-assisted delivery, your doctor may perform a sonogram. He or she will tell you how your labor is progressing and answer your questions.

At this point your doctor will be able to tell you if you're very early in labor and can return home or remain in the hospital waiting area until your labor progresses further.

If your labor has progressed enough, you'll be admitted to the labor suite. This means you are officially in labor. You may be offered an enema to clear out your bowels. The enema is usually not mandatory but can make your delivery more comfortable. They're a good idea if you are frequently constipated or haven't had a bowel movement the day you go into labor. An IV may also be started if there's some concern that you may be dehydrated or need extra energy from the sugar water in the IV.

Assessing How Your Baby Is Doing

When you're admitted to the hospital or birthing center, your doctor will want to know how your baby is doing in this early stage of labor. There are several diagnostic tools that assess your baby's health in the womb.

As discussed in Chapter 6, one of your doctor's most important tools is the *fetal heart monitor*. This will tell your doctor or nurse if the baby's heart rate is within normal range—110 to160 beats per minute. Some change in a baby's heart rate *variability* is normal and expected during labor and delivery, but any significant change in heart rate—such as a steady drop or increase in beats per minute—lets the doctor or nurse know that your baby's condition needs to be monitored more closely. You may be asked to shift your position, take some supplemental oxygen, or have an IV started to offset dehydration. Most of the time, the fetal monitor acts as reassurance that your baby is doing well.

There are two kinds of fetal monitoring. You may have *continuous* (*persistent*) or *periodic* fetal monitoring. Most hospitals use continuous monitoring, and most birthing centers use periodic monitoring. There are two ways to perform continuous fetal heart monitoring: *externally* or *internally*. External fetal heart monitoring is what we have been referring to as nonstress-test (NST) monitoring. External electrodes are attached to the outside of your body with stretchy bands. With internal monitoring, an electrode is inserted into your vagina and attached to your baby's scalp. In order to achieve this, your amniotic sac must be broken, a painless and quick procedure. Another device is inserted inside of your womb to record the strength of contractions. The internal monitoring method is considered more accurate than the external but is more invasive to you and your baby.

Periodic monitoring is called *auscultation,* is a method of listening to the baby's heart rate. It can be done through a *fetoscope*, an instrument similar to a stethoscope that listens for heartbeats. The fetoscope enables your midwife or nurse to hear the fetal heartbeat when pressed to your abdomen. Another device used for auscultation for periodic monitoring is a portable *Doppler*. This is an electronic mechanism that uses sound waves to record the heartbeats. Periodic monitoring is done at regular intervals, at least once every hour throughout labor.

Position and Presentation of the Baby

Your doctor or midwife will also want to determine how your baby is lying in the womb. The baby's position or presentation during labor can influence the type of labor pains you may have (i.e., back labor), the type of delivery you will have (vaginal or cesarean), and usually the length of your labor and delivery. Your midwife or doctor feels the baby's body parts through your abdomen or uses an abdominal sonogram. Most babies are vertex or cephalic, meaning the baby's head is down. Having a baby in the breech or transverse position is one of the common reasons for a cesarean delivery.

The *position* of your baby refers to the way it is facing. The back of the baby's head, the *occiput*, is used to describe the position the baby is facing. Facing toward your back, the anterior position, is most common. Posterior position means your baby is facing your abdomen. Posterior position is usually a major cause of "back labor" because your baby's back is pushing against your backbone. With back labor your contractions are felt mostly in your back rather than your abdomen.

Assessing the size of your baby's head and the position of the placenta gives your doctor or midwife other important clues about how the birth will proceed.

The Baby's Station

The baby's *station* is an estimate of how far down the birth canal your baby has progressed. Knowing the station tells the doctor or midwife how far along the delivery is. The stations start at −5 station and progress backward toward zero and then to +1 to +5 station (see Figure 7-2). At

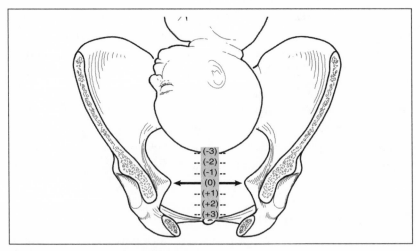

FIGURE 7-2   The fetus at 26 weeks.

zero station, the baby's head is at the level of the *ischial spines*, the bones you can feel on your bottom when you sit on your hands. Zero station is midway through the pelvis and an exciting time because you are close to delivery.

Stages of Labor and Delivery

Labor and delivery is divided into three stages:

1. *The first stage is labor.* Labor is further divided into three phases: early (or latent) active phase, and finally, transition.
2. *The second stage is delivery of the baby.* Delivery is through the vaginal birth canal, or through the abdominal wall with surgery.
3. *The third stage is delivery of the placenta,* or afterbirth. Delivery of the placenta is usually very quick. You can turn all of your attention to your baby.

First Stage

The longest stage of labor is the first. This is when you work the hardest. All of your childbirth preparation is used during this first stage.

In early labor your body slowly gets ready for birth. Your contractions become regular and increase in frequency and length. You may see bloody mucus on your underwear or feel a trickle or strong gush of clear fluid from your vagina. Most of your early labor will be in your home. Generally, early labor is the longest phase of the first stage of labor, and the easiest. Early labor gently makes changes in your cervix and other parts of your body to prepare for birth.

Your goal in early labor is to try to remain as relaxed as possible. Engage in some mild activity that requires you to be upright and standing, such as walking. Ask your doctor or midwife if you can have a light snack with plenty of fluids. You should spend as much time as you can in the comfort of home before going to the hospital or birthing center, but follow your doctor's instructions on when to come to the hospital or birthing center.

Active labor is defined by stronger and more rhythmic contractions. The contractions seem to build and subside like waves, and in most cases are felt over the entire abdomen, not just the lower part. Your uterus is getting down to business and your whole body will feel involved. The goal of active labor is to get your cervix almost completely open, to move the baby into position down in the pelvis, and to stimulate the baby for birth. Your water may break during active labor, or the doctor or midwife may break it with a small hook if she or he feels it might improve labor. Active labor is usually shorter than early labor and is often much more intense.

Your goal during active labor is to allow your body to do its job and to try to relax and conserve energy.

TRY THIS

- Have your partner or doula help you try different positions to minimize the discomfort and to promote relaxing.
- Try to keep moving by getting up to go to the bathroom, walking around the room, and sitting in a chair. Muscles tense when they're held in the same position and will use up oxygen and calories and increase pain.
- Try warm showers and massage.
- Start the breathing and relaxation techniques you learned in your childbirth classes.
- Empty your bladder frequently.
- Sip water or suck on ice chips. You may be allowed Popsicles.

Transition labor is the shortest and most intense part of labor. If you were to liken it to a rafting trip, this would be the roughest "white water." This is when your childbirth preparation—visualization, relaxation, and breathing—is critical. Contractions continue to get stronger, last 60 to 90 seconds, and have almost no pause between them. When the cervix has dilated and effaced to 10 centimeters and the baby's head enters the birth canal, you may feel an increase in pressure on your rectum and lower back. This pressure, along with the very strong contractions, is what makes transition labor uncomfortable. This is called the transition phase because your body transitions from the first, labor stage to the second, delivery stage. This is the shortest phase of labor but also the most challenging because you feel no ability to control your body.

Your goal during transition labor is to keep your focus, conserve energy, and let your body have control and do its job.

TRY THIS

- Panting helps keep you from pushing too early, and breathing exercises distract your mind from the intense contractions.
- Change positions frequently. Try to roll from side to side, sit, or get on your hands and knees on the bed. These changes in position will help relax your muscles and regulate your breathing so you and the baby get more oxygen.
- Put ice packs on your back to relax tense muscles and numb the back pain.
- Keep close contact with your partner or coach. At this point you may want to be left alone to internalize your feelings and pain. Don't let this happen! Prearrange a signal to let your spouse or coach know you're feeling this way. Tell yourself to keep listening to your coach. This is probably the most critical time for your coach to offer encouragement.
- Request something for pain. Talk with your doctor or midwife about this before you go into labor. Know what's available, the degree of relief you can expect, and when and how the medication is given. This is often the time when women request something for pain if they haven't already had an epidural.

You may feel an urge to push as your baby moves down into your pelvis. Your doctor or midwife will tell you when you can begin to push.

Second Stage

When you're in labor, especially the transition phase, you have no concept of time. You just know you're getting tired and don't want to labor anymore. Finally, you hear the magic word, "Complete." Immediately afterward, you'll sense a change in the mood of the room. The doctor or midwife is preparing for the delivery. You may be saying to yourself, "But I feel the same, what's different?" The answer is, your cervix has done its job. You are completely opened up, and now your baby's head can safely come out of the uterus and into the vagina or birth canal. You will be told to push. Pushing helps the baby get lower in the birth canal as quickly as possible.

Delivery

Getting to this stage is wonderful, but you still have work to do. You won't be having very hard contractions, but when they come, you'll need to work with them to push your baby out. Once your baby's head passes the pubic bone, the skin around the perineum—the soft tissue between the anal opening and vaginal opening—will stretch and bulge. The top of your baby's head will be visible through the vaginal opening. Your baby is said to be *crowning*.

Sometimes at this point you and your baby will need a little help. Your doctor or midwife may make an incision in the perineum to ease the strain of the stretched skin and to prevent tearing. This makes the opening larger. The procedure is called an *episiotomy*. Less commonly, your doctor or midwife will carefully place *forceps*—spoon-shaped tongs—into your vagina to grasp the sides of your baby's head or place a *vacuum* device around the top of the baby's head to help your baby out of the birth canal.

When your baby's head emerges, the doctor or midwife will support the head and allow the baby to twist to one side or the other. This frees up the shoulders. Once a shoulder is reachable, slight pressure will be put on the perineum to ease the shoulders out of the birth canal. Once the shoulders are out, the hips and legs usually slide out easily. After your baby is out, contractions decrease in intensity and duration.

Third Stage

The third stage of labor and delivery is the delivery of your placenta, or the "afterbirth." The milder contractions of your uterus cause your placenta to separate from the uterus. You will be asked to give a few more pushes to get the placenta out. Sometimes your doctor or midwife may also need to do some firm massaging of your abdomen to get the uterus to release the placenta. Your placenta is inspected visually and sent to the lab for further evaluation.

Let's take a look at delivery from another's perspective.

   Andy's Story

> *I feel great, so warm and so comfortable. What's that feeling? Feels like someone just gave me a great big hug. I want to hug back but all I can do is kick for joy. These hugs keep happening except they are lasting longer and getting stronger. Yeah out there, I love you too, but you don't have to hug so much. I guess I'll take a nap. Wow, my mom's heartbeat is fast right now. I can tell we are going for a car ride. Hum, I love to kick in the car. The hugging is still going on. Someone is putting something cool on the outside of my mom and now my mom is lying down. The hugging is really getting out of control. I guess I'll kick back so they know I love them too. Whoa, what happened? My bathtub has sprung a leak! I feel myself sliding down. This is exciting; I never did this before. Wow, this tunnel is so tight, I don't know if I can fit. Hey, don't get so pushy. I'm moving. Okay, I passed one corner. Here's another one. You know, I really don't want to play anymore. But I can't seem to go backward. Somebody is touching my head. Hey that feels funny. I feel like I'm being stretched out. Somebody is pulling something over my head. Hey, I see light. I'm kind of getting scared. I'm going to cry. Oh my, what is this? I can see so many things. Hey, what's that? I hear my mom's and dad's voices. I'll be okay now.*

Failure to Progress

Your labor may not proceed steadily to the birth of your baby. "Failure to progress" means your contractions are not preparing your body for delivery. There are several causes. Your contractions may not be strong enough to change your cervix or to help move your baby down into the birth canal. Sometimes you can become so tired that you cannot continue with the labor.

Whatever the reason, when failure to progress occurs, you'll need additional medication to get your contractions going or to make them more intense and effective. This medication, called Pitocin, can only be given in a hospital where you and you baby can be monitored closely. If Pitocin does not get your labor going, you may be allowed to rest a while and try again. If it is still not successful, your doctor will discuss with you the possibility of having a cesarean delivery.

Cesarean Section

Several conditions that arise during pregnancy or during labor may necessitate a delivery by cesarean section (c-section). You may know you have a very strong chance of having a cesarean delivery before going into labor. Your doctor or midwife has been watching your pregnancy all along. Recent examinations may have revealed that your baby seems too large for your pelvis. This is called *cephalo-pelvic-disproportion* (CPD).

Your baby's head might be too large to go through the birth canal, your pelvis shape cannot accommodate a normal size baby's head, or the baby could be in a position that would put strain on its head during birth. Or for other reasons, your doctor may have warned you that a vaginal delivery would be difficult or ill-advised. If you're carrying twins, you already know you are more likely to have a cesarean delivery, and if you're carrying a higher number of multiples, then you are almost certain to have a cesarean delivery.

As mentioned earlier, babies in the breech or transverse position are more likely to be delivered surgically. If you've developed a complication during pregnancy, such as pregnancy induced hypertension or diabetes, your doctor will probably prepare you for the possibility that your baby will arrive by c-section.

Two conditions for cesarean cannot be predicted because they occur after labor is underway. Failure to progress is a common reason for needing a cesarean. Another reason is *fetal distress*, which would be revealed by the fetal monitor. It means your baby is exhibiting signs that he or she is not doing well during labor. If this is the case, the goal is to get your baby delivered quickly and safely.

Most cesareans can be performed using a regional anesthesia, such as an epidural or spinal block. You will be awake for the surgery and your partner can be by your side. Only very rarely does the surgery require general anesthesia. If you do need general anesthesia, you will be asleep and your partner cannot attend the surgery. The procedure is usually so quick that the anesthesia does not affect your baby.

FACTS
The five most common reasons for having a labor end in a cesarean birth are:

- Baby is too large to pass through the vagina and pelvis
- Breech presentation
- Placenta previa
- Failure of the labor to progress
- Cord prolapse (cord around the baby's neck)[3]

Preparation

If your doctor decides your baby should be delivered by cesarean, a team of operating room medical staff will prepare you for surgery. You may be given a medication to dry the secretions in your mouth and upper airway and reduce acid in your stomach. Your pubic and abdominal region will be shaved and cleaned with sterile solution. Usually, a catheter is inserted into the urethra to drain urine. This keeps the bladder empty, so it's unlikely to be injured during the surgery. An IV line will be placed in your arm or hand or wrist to deliver fluids and medications during the surgery. Once you are in the operating room, you'll also have the tubing in place in your back for an epidural or spinal block. Once on the operating table, sterile draping will shield you from a view of the incision.

The Surgery

To perform a cesarean, your obstetrical surgeon will make incisions through your skin, through some other layers of tissue, and finally through the uterus. The uterine incision may be horizontal across the lower part of your abdomen or one of two kinds of vertical cuts. Once the uterine wall is open, your doctor will push down on your uterus just below your chest, to help the baby out of the uterus. This won't hurt but may feel like he or she is pulling on your midsection. Your baby is lifted out and his or her care proceeds as with a vaginal birth. You may be able to stroke your baby while your incision is being closed.

The total surgical event usually takes less than an hour. You will be wheeled to the recovery room and eventually to your hospital room after the doctor repairs your incision. Your vital signs will be checked once you're in the room and every few hours for the next 24-hour period.

Recovery from a Cesarean

The catheter in your bladder will be removed after surgery, but your IV will remain in place for one to two days or until you can take food and drink by mouth. As the anesthesia wears off, you will be very sore and in pain. Your doctor will prescribe pain medication. Let your doctor know if you need more. While you're in the hospital, a nurse will probably show you how to press a pillow into your stomach when getting in and out of bed to minimize the pain. You'll be encouraged to get up frequently. If you've had general anesthesia, you will be encouraged to try to cough up secretions from your lungs.

If you are planning to breast-feed your baby, you'll be encouraged to try nursing your baby. A lactation consultant is usually available, but don't hesitate to ask for guidance from your nurse. Your baby may not latch on easily at first, but try to stick with it. Get help and support with positioning your baby for breastfeeding after a cesarean surgery. As with other kinds of surgery, recovery will take three to four weeks. You should not drive for two weeks. You will be instructed on how to look for signs that your incision may be infected.

Being Postdate

Do you know someone who is almost always late for a meeting or an event? They always get there eventually, but only after much frustration on your part. You may feel irritated with this person. The waiting may make you anxious. Well, this is how you might feel if you haven't given birth and you've passed your due date by two weeks. This is especially difficult if you've had a complicated pregnancy. Through much effort on your part, you've made it to the "finish line" only to find the event isn't over.

Very early in the pregnancy you were told your due date. This is computed by adding 280 days, or 40 weeks, to the first day of your last menstrual period. This date may have been changed by a few days or even a few weeks if an ultrasound led your doctor or midwife to believe your baby was earlier or farther along than indicated by the first due date. When your due date is firmly established, your OB provider expects you will have your baby sometime between the thirty-eighth and forty-second week of your pregnancy. If your baby is not born within the two weeks after your due date, it is considered *postdate*.

After 42 weeks gestation, your doctor or midwife will closely monitor your pregnancy to be sure that the placenta is still functioning effectively to supply nutrition and oxygen to your baby. Other complications that can occur as a result of your baby's overstay in the womb are that your baby may grow too large for a vaginal delivery, or the amount of meconium (the greenish bowel movement of the baby) may increase in the bag of water. The baby would be in danger of inhaling this meconium at the time of delivery. Electronic fetal monitoring, ultrasound, and noting how much your baby kicks will give your OB provider valuable information about how and when to induce labor or plan for a cesarean section delivery.

Induction

If you are postdates, your OB provider may try to artificially induce or start your labor. This is referred to as an *induction*. One method of induction, *stripping the amniotic membranes*, is thought to be effective in getting labor to start or resume and can be done in the OB provider's office. With this procedure, your OB provider sweeps a finger inside the lip of the cervix to pull the membrane away from the wall of the uterus. This action can cause some spotting and cramping. If stripping the amniotic membranes does not help, your doctor will admit you to the hospital and may use the following methods:

- *Cervical ripening* is used to get labor started by dilating and softening your cervix. Medical cervical ripening uses medications that are either swallowed or put into your cervix. *Mechanical cervical ripening* is the insertion of a sterile tube and balloon apparatus into the cervix to stretch the opening.
- A very common method of induction used along with cervical ripening is *administering Pitocin intravenously*. This medication works very effectively to make contractions get stronger to start labor. Some women need this medication throughout the labor and some only once to jump-start the labor.
- Your doctor or midwife may also decide to *rupture your membranes*, using a sterile plastic hook to puncture the amniotic sac. There is no pain, just pressure, but it is thought that the baby's head can move closer to the cervix to help the labor progress.

After Delivery in a Hospital

After a vaginal delivery your baby is quickly inspected by the doctor/midwife and then wrapped in warm blankets and placed on your abdomen while the doctor or midwife place two clamps on the umbilical chord. Sometimes your partner is allowed to cut the cord. After letting you get acquainted, your baby is handed over to a nurse who takes it to a waiting bassinetlike surface for its APGAR tests.

The APGAR test is named for Dr. Virginia Apgar, the physician who developed the scoring system, but it's also an acronym for appearance (color), pulse, grimace (muscle reflex), activity, and respiration. A number value from 1 to 10 tells your baby's pediatrician how your baby did during labor and gives a basic picture of the overall health of your baby just after birth.

APGARs are done at one minute and at five minutes after birth. If your baby is having a problem, there is also an evaluation after 10 minutes. Scores over 7 are good. If your baby has a low score at the five-minute APGAR, he or she will be given immediate care. APGAR is not an intelligence test but simply a score of how your baby is doing at birth.

Once the APGARs are done, your baby can be returned to you. If you'd like to try, you can attempt nursing. Your nurse will put identically numbered bracelets on you and your baby. Warm blankets will be wrapped around the baby and a hat will help hold in heat. Later, when you're getting ready to go back to a postpartum room, your baby will be taken to a nursery to be bathed, dried, weighed, and measured.

You may get chills after delivery. This is normal. The dampness of the gown you're wearing and the fact that you have suddenly stopped working hard can cause you to feel cold. The nurse will bring you warmed blankets. She'll check your blood pressure and temperature and provide you with a sanitary napkin to absorb the bleeding. Your uterus will be checked for firmness.

After your baby has nursed or when you're tired, the baby will be taken to the nursery unless you request that it remain in the room with you. You'll probably remain in the hospital for a day or two.

After Delivery in a Birthing Center

Postdelivery care is similar in a birthing center, but the policy of midwives is to interrupt the family bonding as little as necessary. Because babies remain in the birthing room with their mothers, there is no need to put matching bracelets on mother and baby for identification. Your midwife will stay with you until your vital signs are stable.

If you deliver at a birthing center, you and the midwife will discuss when you and the baby can go home. The usual stay is 6 to 12 hours after birth, but this can vary with each mother and each center. Many birthing center mothers are anxious to get home to their own beds and do not find the short stay unsettling.

Bonding

The bond between you and your baby, and between your partner and your baby, begins the moment you lay eyes on each other, smell each other, and feel each other's skin. It's a sensory experience. There is really nothing you have to do but *be with your infant*. While you're using your senses to get to know your new baby, your baby is doing the same with you. In scientific terminology, this is called *imprinting*. You are memorizing each other.

Imprinting, or bonding, can begin whenever the three of you are able to be together. Your baby may need immediate medical attention and be whisked away to the nursery or NICU. You may have had a cesarean delivery or a very difficult labor and delivery and need some time to recuperate. You may not be able to hold your baby immediately after delivery. Don't worry, bonding will still occur when you two can be together.

Immediately Postpartum

The immediate concern of the nurses is to check your uterus to make sure it is firm. Firmness indicates that any blood vessels opened during the delivery are closing off. Your nurse or midwife may massage your uterus periodically (every few hours). This *fundal massage* keeps the uterus firm and prevents excessive blood loss. You can ask them to teach you how to do this. You'll also probably experience some after-birth cramps. This is a good thing since it means the uterus is working to expel any remaining tissues and get your uterus back to shape.

Postdelivery bleeding—the *lochia*—will be very heavy and probably bright red in color. There may be clots for the first few days. They should get smaller in size and become less frequent. Gradually over the next two to three days, the lochia should change to a dark color like a menstrual period and the clots should disappear.

Going Home

You may have a quick labor or a long one, have pain medication or go without, have a vaginal birth or a cesarean, have an early, on time, or late baby. However your delivery goes, you'll be bringing home your newborn baby. You've done it. Having a baby is a huge accomplishment. You will be able to congratulate yourself for how well you took care of yourself during your pregnancy, how well you prepared for labor and delivery, and how you persevered during the arduous hours of contractions. You should also plan to forgive yourself for anything you did or didn't do during the pregnancy, labor, and delivery. Rest assured, OB practitioners and their staff have seen and heard it all.

Before you leave the hospital or birthing center, make sure you understand when to make a follow-up appointment for yourself and a first pediatrician appointment for your newborn. Most pediatricians want to meet your baby the day after you get home and again at two weeks of age. You will probably be asked to schedule an appointment with your doctor to return at or before six weeks after the birth. Be ready to tell him or her what kind of birth control you plan to use.

Once you get home, it will be time to celebrate, restore your strength, and get to know your baby. Your pregnancy journey will be just about complete. Your "raising a child" journey is just getting started. The next chapter wraps up any of the loose ends of your pregnancy journey. This final part of your adventure is the postpartum period.

In the unsettled time after you come back home, try to take a few minutes to write down everything you remember about the birth of your baby. Have your partner write his recollections as well, since he'll have a different perspective. It may seem like the two of you will never forget any of it, but unfortunately, you probably will. If you've written it all down, you'll have a document to share with your child when he or she grows up. Our own children still clamor for retellings of their births. Yours will too.

8

Your Postpartum Period

 Danielle's Journal

> *Dear Journal,*
> *Amelia was born at 2:05 a.m. and weighed six pounds, one ounce. She's so perfect. When she's awake, she seems to know us. I'm so physically tired but also exhilarated. I must be a sight, but Darryl keeps telling me I look beautiful. I wanted to nurse right after the delivery, but we didn't really get the hang of it. We tried again later, and it seemed to go a little better. It doesn't matter, we have our baby. I can't believe she's really here!*

After you've had some time with your newborn, perhaps tried to nurse and made a few phone calls to spread the happy news, it's time for you to eat, drink, and go to sleep. Most hospitals and all birthing centers allow the baby to stay with you after delivery. However, you'll need to rest and so will your baby. Both of you have worked really hard over the past few days. Your partner may be tired too. You can put the baby in a bassinet near your bed and take a nap. Or your partner or the special person you invited to attend the birth can hold your baby while you sleep. If you are in the hospital, you can have the nurse take the baby to the nursery if you prefer. Sleep is a powerful restorative.

After a rest or nap, you may begin to notice how your body has changed. You may even miss feeling the baby's movements. Your abdomen will have shrunk, but you may still look six or seven months pregnant. Your figure will dramatically improve with time. One of the fastest ways to get it back in shape is to breast-feed, which we'll get to shortly.

Breast-Feeding at the Hospital

If you choose, after delivery and some rest, you can get started breast-feeding, or continue your efforts if you have already begun. Your first attempt after you and your baby have rested may be more successful than when you initially tried. Your baby may be feeling hungry enough to work at breast-feeding a little longer.

Ask your doula, midwife, or nurse to help you with breast-feeding, or request a *lactation consultant*—usually a nurse who has special training in breast-feeding. Most hospitals provide this service. She can help you with "latching on" and nursing in different positions, which will help you avoid sore nipples.

Breast-feeding takes motivation and practice. Any anxiety you feel about nursing will be greatly reduced if you can get your baby to nurse successfully in the hospital or birthing center. In addition, this early nursing will give him or her high-calorie, high-protein *colostrum*, the clear breast milk that helps protect your baby from infections and disease for the first six months.

If you don't feel that both of you have gotten the hang of it by the time you can go home, it's still not too late. Ask for follow-up coaching over the phone or a meeting with a lactation consultant in their office or in your home. Sometimes this is covered by your insurance. Breast-feeding is good for you and your baby. It's worth persevering.

The Day After Delivery

If you had a vaginal delivery, by the second day you will feel pain and swelling in your *perineum,* the opening to your vagina. You may also feel pain and soreness from your stitches if you've had an episiotomy. The discomfort may make it uncomfortable to sit down. Analgesic pain medication should alleviate this discomfort, but the best method is to try soaking twice a day or more in a shallow warm tub bath—called a "sitz bath." The warm water sooths the area, promotes healing, and keeps the area clean. You can also try squirting warm water over the affected area with a *peri bottle* while sitting on the toilet. A peri bottle is simply a plastic bottle with a squirt top and is often provided by the hospital or birthing center. You should continue this practice at home until your stitches are healed.

If you delivered by cesarean section, your abdomen may have a three to four-inch incision, which may be a little swollen and uncomfortable at first. Pain from the surgery that usually requires pain medication will occur in the next few days. As your spinal or epidural anesthesia wears off, you may notice a backache and/or headache. Your IV will be left in to provide you with antibiotics if needed and/or fluids until you can drink without feeling sick to your stomach. The bladder catheter will be removed as soon as the anesthesia has worn off and you can stand. You should have assistance the first time you get up to go to the bathroom since you'll probably be unsteady on your feet. Try pressing a pillow into your middle when getting out of bed, to ease your abdominal discomfort.

If you had general anesthesia, you'll be encouraged to get out of bed for short periods as soon as possible. This will prevent lung congestion and any other complications of general anesthesia. You will also be asked to try to take deep breaths and cough or use a breathing machine to help clear your lungs and prevent pneumonia.

As with other kinds of surgery, recovery from a cesarean may take three to four weeks. You may be advised not to drive for two weeks. Once home, you can shower, and many OB providers say it's okay to take tub baths. Check with him or her on this prior to being discharged from the hospital. You will probably be asked to return in two weeks to make sure the incision is healing. You should know the signs and symptoms of an infection and who and when to call if you develop these symptoms. These symptoms include fever greater than 100º F by mouth, chills, pain in your abdomen or at the incision site, and redness or swelling at the incision site.

While you're still surrounded by medical expertise, *ask as many questions as you can about your recovery and the care of your baby.* Be sure you know what to look for when you get home, what's normal and what could be a problem.

Arriving Home

By day five most new moms are home with their babies. Your immediate task is to take care of yourself and your baby, continue to rest, eat, and drink to regain your strength and heal. You'll also be using this time to get to know your baby. Your partner's task is to rest, take care of all of you, and the baby, and help you get the rest you need.

When your baby is only 2–5 days old, you'll probably make your first expedition out with your new baby to his or her initial visit to the pediatrician. Your pediatrician will already have the OB provider's delivery report, your baby's record from the hospital, and any other important discharge information. A physical exam, height and weight measurement, another PKU test, and perhaps some vaccinations for your baby will be part of this first visit. Use the opportunity to ask questions about your baby's behavior, feeding, and health.

Your immediate days at home will probably be taken up with adjusting to your baby, particularly his or her sleep patterns. Your baby may sleep for anywhere between two to four hours at a time during the day or night. Most babies don't sleep longer than four hours because their stomachs can only fill with enough milk to last a 2–4 hour period. They will awaken when they are hungry again. Thus, it's likely that your own sleep patterns will be the same as your baby's. So try to fight the urge to stay awake and visit or clean house; instead, take naps when your baby does. *Rest is very important during your recovery* and to help with successful breast-feeding. Listen to your body when it's telling you it needs rest. Many pediatricians recommend going with whatever schedule occurs during the first week or so, realizing that the baby will probably sleep longer when it gets a little older.

Try to get help for meals and household responsibilities from family members or a close friend or neighbor the first week after getting home or plan on preparing meals ahead of time that just need to be warmed up and let the housework go. Later your partner can take on most of the household chores so you can attend to the baby and sleep. You'll probably feel up to answering phone calls and receiving a few guests who want to congratulate you and meet your baby, but have your helper or partner be the gatekeeper, protecting you from calls and visits when you're resting. Most people are sensitive to making sure you get your rest, especially if they've had babies and remember how tiring that first week home was.

Breast Care after Delivery

At the beginning of Chapter 7, we reviewed the pros and cons of breast-feeding and bottle-feeding. By now you have probably decided which method you want to start out with. However, it is helpful to know how to care for your breasts after you have a baby.

About three to five days after you've had the baby, your breast milk will "come in." This means the colostrum is now replaced with breast milk. If you are nursing, you may feel liquid moving quickly through your breast or you may notice that the breast your baby is not nursing from is leaking fluid. This is called the "let-down reflex." The let-down reflex often occurs when your baby cries to be fed.

During this same time, you'll feel as if you have two hard heavy balls on your chest. Your breasts are *engorged* or swollen with breast milk, whether you plan to breast-feed or not. This is a normal function of the breast, but it can be uncomfortable, especially if you do not plan to breast-feed. The solution to this problem is basically the same regardless of what your feeding plans are. To decrease the discomfort from engorgement you can:

- Check your temperature and your breast for signs of an infection. Call your OB provider if your temperature is over 100º F by mouth, if your breasts become extremely hard, or if the skin is pinkish-red and hot to the touch like a sunburn. You may have an infection of the breast called *mastitis* that can be treated with antibiotics. Wear a bra that fits snugly. The pressure will work against the discomfort. If you are breast-feeding wear a comfortable and supportive nursing bra.
- Take warm showers. These will soften the breast tissue and expel some milk. If you are breast-feeding, try to expel some milk before you try feeding the baby. When your breasts are very hard, your baby has a harder time latching onto a nipple to nurse. Getting the flow started will help soften the breast and allow the baby to nurse. If you are bottle-feeding don't pump your breasts. Pumping stimulates increased production of milk.
- Put ice packs on your breasts. The cold reduces blood supply to your breasts. Reduced blood supply decreases milk production

and alleviates the pain and swelling. If you are breast-feeding do this after nursing.

- Check with your OB provider about taking analgesics like Tylenol or Advil.
- If you're planning to breast-feed, use a pad of cotton inside the bra cup to catch leaking milk. This will keep you from having to change your clothes as often. Try to get plenty of fluids, rest, and eat healthy food and find out what resources are available to get continuing professional support. The critical time to get help is when you first get home; the support and advice of a lactation expert can improve your chances of continuing to breast-feed.

Minor Aches and Pain After Delivery

- Your bleeding will continue to be bright red with a few small clots after you get home, but the bleeding should decrease in amount and darken to a brownish color, and the clots will diminish. You should continue to massage your uterus for the next few days to help it release the clots and decrease your bleeding. Let your doctor know if you have a sudden increase in lochia that is bright red in color and you are using more than one pad an hour.
- You may feel "after birth" pains while you are nursing or are just relaxing—sharp gaslike pains or cramping. This is caused by your uterus contracting as it decreases in size.
- Your perineum will be sore and slightly swollen. The sitz baths mentioned above will help with this discomfort and promote healing of small tears or stitches.
- Your back may ache from the delivery or the epidural. Try a heating pad or warm water from a shower or bath and acetaminophen (Tylenol) if needed.
- You may notice swollen or sore hemorrhoids. These are varicose veins in the rectum that usually result from the weight of the uterus or the forceful pushing during delivery of your baby. Sitz baths will also alleviate the discomfort of hemorrhoids, along with medicated sprays, ointments, or pads. A diet high

in fiber is important to prevent constipation and promote healing of hemorrhoids. Talk to your OB provider if you think
something isn't right or you feel your body isn't recovering
expected. A telephone call can relieve stress and worry.

Eating Well After the Delivery

The number of times your newborn wakes to be fed or changed is
likely to cause fatigue, so catching up on sleep may feel more important than eating and drinking. For the same reason, you might not
pay attention to what, or even if, you are eating, and you may have
lost your appetite. To counter this, get something to eat and drink
every time you feed your baby, this means you may be snacking every
3–4 hours. Make sure the selection of food you choose is good for you
and your baby's health.

Your diet is very important to your recovery, and it's critical if you're
breast-feeding your baby, since it means you'll need more calories than
you needed during pregnancy. These extra calories should come from
nutritious food, not from fats and sugars. It's also a good idea to stay
away from fried, spicy, greasy, or gas-producing foods, since these can
upset both your and your baby's systems. Ask your partner or support
person to tempt you with delicious and, more important, nutritious
meals and snacks.

You should also keep yourself well hydrated. Have a bottle or glass
of water nearby every time you nurse. This will help you produce more
breast milk if you are nursing and help prevent constipation. Your diet
and fluid intake play an important role in giving you the strength and
vitality to recover from the delivery and take care of yourself and your
baby in these first few weeks.

Sometimes even if you are getting plenty of sleep, good food, and
water, you may become constipated. Try increasing your intake of fiber
by eating at least *two servings of bran per day*. Bran comes in cereals,
muffins, and waffles. There is also a powdered form you can add to
casseroles or soups. Prunes or other dried fruits may also help with your
irregularity, but they can cause uncomfortable gas. If you feel you
need a laxative, get approval from your doctor or midwife first.

Fatigue

The most common complaint about recovering from a birth and caring for a newborn is the overwhelming fatigue. Most parents simply cannot believe how tired they are, and they wonder how long they can continue getting broken sleep. Happily, newborn "boot camp" doesn't usually last long for most families.

Here are some tips on fighting fatigue:

- Start gentle exercises and stretches. Even five minutes of stretching several times a day is beneficial. This will relax you and ease muscle strain. Avoid doing exercises just before bedtime at night, as this activity may simulate you and cause wakefulness.
- Cut down or cut out caffeinated beverages like tea, coffee, cola, and chocolate. They may be keeping you up at the wrong times or, worse, keeping your baby up.
- Fight the urge to stay up and clean or do other things when your baby is sleeping. The rule in the immediate postpartum period is to sleep or quietly rest when your baby does.
- Get help from your partner, your family, and friends. Encourage family and friends to bring meals when they visit or help with weekly chores like laundry or grocery shopping. Don't be shy about asking for help. Most will be thrilled to be of service.
- One or two days out of the week, let your partner get up and bottle-feed the baby with pumped breast milk or formula. This will give you a longer stretch of uninterrupted sleep. If your partner is also exhausted, ask a friend or relative to spend the night. An occasional bottle-feeding without you will not harm your baby, but wait to start this until your breast-feeding is well established.

Being Alone with Your Baby

Eventually, it will be time for family members or friend to return home, and your partner to return to work. You'll be alone with your baby. At first it may be a relief to have some time alone with your baby at home. This time may help you and your baby get into more of a routine and maybe give you more time to sleep. But your home can get very quiet. And the quiet may only be punctuated by the screams of your baby trying to communicate some discomfort.

You may feel uncomfortable in this new circumstance, especially if you had a very fast-paced, people-filled life prior to the birth of your baby. Try to keep this phase of your life in perspective. You will never have this time with your baby again. He or she will get older and more independent and you will have other needs pulling you in other directions. Relish this "just the two of you" time, document it with photos, journals, and recordings.

You may still feel the need to schedule events to break up the time alone. Get out the baby stroller and take walks, weather permitting, or arrange to meet with other new moms you may have met during your childbirth preparation class or with coworkers. Call friends, to talk, ask questions, and get reassurance. Your baby will be sleeping a lot. Use this time to rest but if you feel rested, consider taking on small projects such as thank-you notes, birth notices, or planning a christening party or other baby-welcoming event. If these sound overwhelming, it's too soon to start doing these activities. Pace yourself. You're having to adjust to this new life with your baby, and you are still recovering from nine months of pregnancy, labor, and delivery.

Postpartum Blues

About 70 to 80 percent of new mothers experience what's often called "postpartum blues."[1] This can last from a couple of days to a couple of weeks, and sometimes will occur one to two months after giving birth. Researchers believe that it's caused by a combination of fatigue and the rapidly changing hormone levels in the body.

Symptoms of postpartum blues include:

- Feeling sad or lonely
- Crying easily
- Mood swings such as happiness and then fear, or sadness and then anger
- Restlessness, irritability, or anxiousness about everything
- Feeling overwhelmed
- Having doubts about how well you're caring for your newborn
- Feeling generally unsatisfied

If you get the blues, you might be astonished that you don't feel completely satisfied about being a mother or about the beautiful baby in front of you. Many times it's because you're expecting too much of yourself too soon. However, be forewarned that your partner and friends may be puzzled and seem unsympathetic if they find you crying over what seems to be trivial matters.

Though scientists point to fatigue and hormones for these baby blues, there may be other factors at work. For one thing, you have just completed a major change in your life, and individuals respond to change differently. You now have a new life with new requirements and new expectations. You literally have a new appearance and a new relationship with your partner. Letting go of the old you may be harder than you thought.

Secondly, no one quite realizes how much work a new baby is until they have one, and by then, of course, there's no going back. It's understandable that you may feel trapped in a new role that at times seems overwhelming. In addition, the fatigue and hormonal changes can magnify underlying problems such as the lack of support from family or friends, a difficult, colicky baby, a fearful partner, or unexpected difficulties with breast-feeding.

It's easy to feel disappointed that gracefully juggling being a mother, wife, and accomplished individual isn't a snap. For the most part, these blues are normal and will fade with time and rest. In the meanwhile, if you or your partner notices that you're unhappy or blue, try the following:

- Let your partner and others know what's going on with you and when you have these feelings.
- Get more rest. This may mean letting the housecleaning go, being late on thank-you notes for the baby gifts, and eating frozen dinners or takeout food more often. If letting things go adds to your stress, try telling yourself that this lowering of your standards is temporary or get help from family and friends.
- Eat healthy meals, without alcohol or other depressants, or stimulants.
- Get out of the house at least once a day and be around others.
- Take time for yourself. Even a half an hour to soak in the tub or polish your nails will refresh you.

- Watch a comedy on TV or listen to one on the radio—laughter is a great mood enhancer.
- Contact hotlines and support groups to get the help you need.
- Let your doctor know if you're not getting better or if you're feeling worse.

Postpartum Depression

If any of the symptoms of the "blues" described above lasts longer than two weeks, you may be suffering from *postpartum depression*. Postpartum depression is a mental health condition that lasts longer than the "blues" and is more disabling to the mother. It is more likely to occur if you have a history of depression, have had postpartum depression after an earlier pregnancy, or have recently experienced an extraordinary life event such as the loss of a job, home, or loved one. It can also occur for no apparent reason. The symptoms of postpartum depression include:

- Feeling sad, unworthy, guilty, or miserable.
- Crying a lot or feeling very angry.
- Feeling alone, excessively worried, scared, anxious, or panicky that you're going to do something wrong or that something bad is going to happen.
- Feeling so tired that you have no energy to take care of your baby or yourself.
- Having trouble enjoying anything or focusing on anything. You feel nothing really matters. You just want to be left alone.
- Being afraid of hurting your baby or yourself.
- Having problems sleeping or a poor appetite, or both.

In fact, postpartum depression may require medication, mental health therapy, or both. The good news is that it is treatable and treatment has good success rates. If you have any of the symptoms just listed, talk to your OB provider immediately. Ask for a referral to a mental health care provider who specializes in postpartum depression. You may be referred to a psychiatrist who can prescribe antidepressants, if these are warranted. Newer kinds of antidepressants are harmless to a breast-fed baby. Remember: this is an illness, not something you caused. You shouldn't feel guilty or ashamed. Get professional help. Your family needs you to get better.

Health Insurance Coverage

Although sensational cases related to postpartum depression have raised public awareness on this topic, many insurance policies do not recognize it as a psychiatric illness and therefore limit treatment coverage. Of course, if you feel you have postpartum depression, do not hesitate to get help. Let your doctor know your concerns about being able to pay for therapy. She or he may be able to write you a referral that will mean psychiatric treatment is covered by your insurance. Many communities have support groups for women with postpartum depression.

You Need to Exercise

It probably seems unrealistic to suggest that you begin to exercise immediately after you have a baby, but this will help you during this recovery phase and get you used to a routine thereafter. It's the best "medicine" you could possibly give yourself to make you feel better.

Try to think of exercise as a way of giving yourself some personal time. Slowly get back to your exercise routine, or start exercising if you weren't doing it before. You'll feel better emotionally and physically, and this will encourage you to continue getting your post-pregnancy body back in shape, you'll feel less tired, and you'll feel better while caring for your baby. Regular exercise improves muscle tone and, more important, creates a feeling of well-being. You'll also be in better shape to carry your baby as he or she starts growing, getting larger and heavier every day.

There are long-term benefits as well. Your baby needs you a lot right now, but he or she will continue to need you in evolving ways for the next 18 years or more. Indeed, your children will greatly benefit from your being around and healthy even after they attain adulthood.

When to Start

Ask your OB/GYN Provider when you can resume exercising, when you should start, and how much exercise is advisable. If you had any complications with your pregnancy, you may be advised to wait a little longer than after an uncomplicated pregnancy.

If you exercised regularly before and during pregnancy, you'll probably feel that you can begin again fairly soon after the delivery. Still, you may want to start with slow walks to gradually get back to your previous level of fitness and get used to your new body. If you're not used to regular exercise, start off slowly but do start exercising. Walking is a good way to get some gentle exercise, without thinking of it as work. Bring the baby along for the fresh air and your partner or a friend for company.

Slow, easy stretching is a form of exercise you can do fairly soon after giving birth that can be done in your home, without classes or cost, and at any time of the day. Many health and fitness clubs, hospitals, and community centers offer postpartum exercise classes, including yoga for new mothers. If you're unsure about what you want to do, you may want to enroll in one of these specially designed classes. The instructor can make sure you're doing the exercises correctly and at an appropriate level of exertion and you'll have a dedicated time to exercise.

You'll probably think of a million reasons why you don't have the time to start an exercise routine, and many are no doubt valid. If you notice that you're watching television instead, use that time to stretch out. You can keep the exercises and stretches described below near the TV. Get on the floor and do them for at least 15 to 20 minutes to start off.

You need to incorporate exercising into your life the way you've incorporated other daily tasks, like brushing your teeth. You deserve to feel good, get back into shape, and improve your ability to relax and sleep better. The most important thing you can do is get moving!

Postpartum Exercises

Try the following exercises after getting approval from your OB/GYN provider. Wear loose clothing, a supportive bra, and have plenty of water nearby for frequent drinks. You should warm up with some walking and cool down with gentle stretches. If anything hurts, stop doing it and talk with your OB provider. Don't do too much your first few times. You may get sore and not want to do them again.

- *Leg stretches.* Lie on your back with your legs bent and feet flat on the floor. Make sure your lower back is not arched away from the floor, but gently making contact with it. Tilt your pelvis to be sure it touches the floor. Slide one leg out until it's straight, and then return it to its bent leg position. Sliding the leg out will make the back arch slightly. Try to work against this. Repeat on the other leg and work to increase your repetitions. As you get stronger, you may also slide the leg out one or two inches above the ground. Be sure your lower back is flat against the floor. Repeat several times with each leg.
- *Pelvic tilt.* On your hands and knees, with your back straight, work to tilt your pelvis forward so your lower back feels rounded, like a cat arching. At the same time, tighten your thigh and buttocks muscles and pull your pubic bone forward toward your head instead of parallel to the floor. It's best to be exhaling while you tilt your pelvis and inhaling as you return to the flat-backed position. This exercise works your hips, thighs, and abdominal muscles. Start off with 5 to 10 of these and increase your number of repetitions gradually.
- *Curls.* This is a progressive exercise. As you get stronger, you gradually work toward the more difficult curls. (As you start, put your hands on your abdomen to remind yourself to pull your stomach in. This keeps you from stretching the gap between your two abdominal muscles.) On your back with your knees bent and feet flat on the floor, lift your head as you exhale. Hold for a moment and lower your head to the floor. When you can do these easily, lift farther, taking your shoulders off the floor; and then, when you can easily do this, lift your upper body off the floor. You reach forward with your arms to lift you higher. Increase the number of repetitions as you get stronger.
- *Kegels, or pelvic-floor muscle exercises.* In any comfortable position, contract your muscles in the lower pelvic area—the muscles you would use to stop a flow of urine. Hold for as long as 10 seconds and slowly release. Do 10 to 20 of these several times a day. It may be easier to remember to do these just after you go to the bathroom.

- *Shoulder shrug.* Your upper back may get sore from curving your shoulders in during nursing or from holding your baby. Try to sit or stand upright. While nursing, place a bed pillow on your lap for the baby to lie on to minimize curving your shoulders in or arching your back. To ease upper body soreness, lift your shoulders toward your ears and let them drop gently, exhaling as you do. Repeat this several times. Then alternate shoulders.
- *Shoulder circles.* Lift your shoulders toward your ears and consciously circle them toward your back. Remember to breathe into the stretch. Do several circles, and repeat the circles in the opposite direction with the shoulders coming forward. Then alternate each shoulder forward and backward.
- *Arm circles.* Lift your arms straight out from your sides at shoulder height and make small circles forward and then back. Do this several times.
- *Back, thigh, and arm stretch. Standing straight, lace your* fingers together behind your back. Squeeze the muscles around your shoulder blades and open up your chest. You can also bend over at the waist very slowly, with knees bent, and pull your arms up toward the ceiling to get a better stretch. This widens your chest and stretches your upper back muscles. Do several repetitions.

Birth Control After Giving Birth

Doctors and midwives usually recommend that you abstain from sexual intercourse for two weeks after delivery and preferably for six weeks. This gives your body a chance to return to normal functioning, allows stitches to heal, and prevents infections and discomfort. Usually, at your six-week checkup, your doctor will ask you what kind of birth control you'd like to use. Review your options beforehand so you'll have an answer in time for this visit. In the meanwhile, plan to have condoms or contraceptive sponges on hand, just in case you decide to have sex sooner than the six-week period. Some women do get pregnant before their six-week checkup.

Choosing a new birth control method will depend on several factors: your current situation, your medical history, your plans for having other

202 Protect Your Pregnancy

children, and the effectiveness of your previous method of birth control. Your last pregnancy may have been an accident. About half of all pregnancies in the United States are unplanned.[2] You know whether you used your previous birth control correctly and consistently. In any case, your situation is different now because you have a young baby to care for. You want a reliable birth control method so you can plan your family.

Sexual Relations After Giving Birth

Some couples are ready to resume sexual relations or love-making as soon as the doctor gives the go ahead, other couples, particularly the new mother, worry about discomfort after having a baby. Fatigue and stress may also influence how you feel about making love. And in some cases, you may be concerned about getting pregnant too soon. Talk to your partner and your OB provider about all of your concerns.

The truth of the matter is, finding the time to make love may be more of a challenge after having a baby, but can be just as enjoyable as before and maybe even better. Find a time when the baby is napping so as not to be interrupted. You may want to have a warm shower and a small glass of wine to relax you. Try activities that will get you more in the mood such as massaging each other. Be aware that you may have some bloody discharge for several weeks after delivery but this is normal as long as you are not having any pain during intercourse. Your breasts may also leak during intercourse or sexual excitement because of your changed hormone levels. Try not to let these changes discourage you. You may want to inform your partner of these possible differences to reassure him. The goal is to just enjoy each other and have no other expectations.

Applaud Yourself

Finally, take the time to enjoy your new life and applaud yourself for your accomplishment. Recognize the good parts as well as the not-so-good. You may be tired and feel misshapen, you may have a messy house, but what's really important is that you have a beautiful baby to cuddle and care for. Take care of yourself so you can take care of your new family member!

9

Prescription:
Activity Reduction and Bed Rest

 Yvonne's Journal

Dear Journal,
    No one at work can believe I'm lying on the sofa, reading books on pregnancy and trying to decide on what boy's name to pike. I, the type A of the group, the one who is the first and the last in the office, am now at a standstill. I tired to convincemy doctor I needed to be back to work. but Dr. Karm showed me photos of a baby born at 28 weeks. That's where I was in my pregnancy when the PIH was discovered. It's been three weeks now, and I know I can do this for my baby. It's about him and his future health.

Bed rest or activity reduction at home is often prescribed if you develop a condition during pregnancy that could lead to premature birth, such as pregnancy-induced hypertension or multiple episodes of preterm labor. Common conditions that often lead to bed rest include:

- Pregnancy-induced hypertension
- Vaginal bleeding
- Preterm premature rupture of membranes
- Carrying twins or triplets
- Intrauterine growth restricted (IUGR) in the baby
- Cervical changes (beginning to dilate and efface) and preterm labor

Bed rest is a prescription for assisting your body to rest in hopes of minimizing the symptoms caused by complications in your pregnancy.

The goal of bed rest is to give your baby more time in the womb until he or she can safely be born.

If you're experienceing complications for unknown reasons, you may fret and worry about "what you did wrong" in your pregnancy to have it be considered high risk and necessitate bed rest.

In the majority of cases ...you didn't do anything wrong!

What's surprising to many women who need bed rest is that they do not feel sick. Some have never felt better. In fact, the bed rest is not primarily for you—it's for your baby.

If you are prescribed bed rest, your doctor is usually expecting you to stop everything that could be physically demanding: work, travel, vacations, family celebrations, *everything*, and stay completely or partially off your feet resting on the couch or in bed. This may be for a few days, weeks, and, in some cases, months. It is not an easy thing for anyone to do. But it can be done, and many women are doing it right now.

You will want to learn what will help you manage this unexpected change in your pregnancy. There are people who want you to succeed—health care professionals, women who have experienced this kind or pregnancy, family and friends. You can work with them to provide your baby the healthiest start in life.

Is Bed Rest Effective?

There's a range of opinions regarding bed rest. Most obstetric providers believe it is beneficial in some cases, although most agree that following the prescription is not easy and not without some side effects.

Bed rest was first prescribed in England in the 1920s when a British physician noticed that twins born to middle-class women were larger and healthier than those born to working-class women. The physician hypothesized that a more leisurely lifestyle was responsible and began placing working-class women carrying twins on bed rest at 32 weeks gestation. In the succeeding years, the practice expanded to include women who experience preterm labor for unknown reasons or develop complications in their pregnancies. Bed rest can be accompanied by tocolytics, medications that try to calm the uterus and stop contractions.

In the United States, most physicians prescribe bed rest when a pregnancy threatens to end prematurely. In hindsight, many women feel they would not have maintained their pregnancies to term if they had not been on bed rest, at home or in the hospital, and many of their doctors agree. But the benefits of bed rest are not well documented in U.S. medical literature, and in fact there have been studies that reveal problems.

In France, a leading researcher in obstetrics, Dr. Papernik, has done a number of clinical studies on the benefits of bed rest for women in preterm labor and for women who are expecting twins. Most of his studies, done with women at home on bed rest, have found that increased rest alone is by and large beneficial. Most U.S. studies, in contrast, involve women who are hospitalized, and some argue that the hospital setting increases stress for the at-risk mother and may lead to more negative results. It's clear that more studies are needed to document whether there truly is any benefit to bed rest, either at home or in the hospital and to the benefits of increased rest for an at-risk pregnancy.

What Does It Accomplish?

Some physicians feel there's a benefit in prescribing bed rest because they feel it tends to slow or stop contractions for some women. The reasons for this are probably because:

- While you're in a horizontal position or sitting up with your legs elevated, less weight is bearing down on the cervix, the opening the baby will pass through in delivery. Circumventing the natural pull of gravity is thought to help prevent preterm labor.
- Lying down helps lower blood pressure, primarily because being horizontal decreases stress on the heart and blood vessels, which don't need to work as hard as when you're upright.
- You are less active, reducing physical stress on your body.
- Decreasing your activity level may decrease blood supply demand from other parts of your body , and thus increase blood supply to the uterus and baby. Therefore, more oxygen will be getting to your baby and your uterus. Conversely, any reduction in the amount of oxygen available to your baby or uterus may cause contractions.
- Increasing your blood supply with bed rest or reduced activity may also increase blood flow to your baby, improving the supply

of nutrients, particularly when your baby is felt to have problems of slow growth (IUGR).

- If you have placenta previa, your placenta is covering the opening of the cervix and has started to bleed. Bed rest may keep the pressure of the baby's head off the placenta and prevent further bleeding.

The Case Against It

As mentioned above, the medical literature in the United States does not always support the benefits of bed rest. It's not universally accepted that bed rest is a recommended method to prevent a possible premature delivery.

In the past 10 years there's been increasing controversy regarding the benefits of bed rest. Some researchers believe that bed rest—especially *strict bed rest*—can cause major complications such as decreased muscle tone, bone loss from calcium depletion, and, in rare situations, possible blood clots. Documented unpleasant side effects of hospital bed rest include leg muscle atrophy and weight loss. It may also cause stress because of separation from family, and some believe it leads to or exacerbates depression. Other reported side effects could also occur with women who are not on bed rest. However, side effects such as heartburn, reflux, headache, and constipation do seem to be more frequent in bed rest patients.

In a study on home bed rest, women reported anxiety, depression, and an inability to stick to the prescription. They felt they had to get up to do things around the home or for themselves, or they believed it was safe to get up more than prescribed. For this reason many physicians prescribe bed rest only for women who absolutely need it, and tailor the amount of resting they have to do according to how well the pregnancy is going.

Initially, Bed Rest or Activity Reduction May Increase Stress

Having to suddenly change from a full-time productive member of a working team to that of being home in bed or off your feet all day, not working, is very stressful. You may worry that you've left co-workers and your boss in the lurch, and you may be anxious that you won't have a job to come back to. If you have other children at home, you may be anxious about finding and affording child care and allaying their anxieties about your not being available to them.

Any and all of these factors can increase your stress at least initially as you try to reorganize work activities, house management, and the care of other children—all in the face of concern about the well-being of your unborn baby. Deciding to focus on the health of your unborn baby may help you realize these other priorities are really less important.

Staying off Your Feet, or Bed Rest

Modern medical science has not yet found a good alternative to bed rest. If you experience preterm labor, you will most likely be told to curtail activity to one degree or another. Your prescription for activity reduction will be designed for your specific situation. In other words, your doctor may feel you need bed rest now but may allow you to return to full activity later in your pregnancy, or may feel that your condition does not warrant bed rest, even when compared to someone who might have similar symptoms.

Your doctor will explain the degree of activity reduction including bed rest that you need to follow, what effects it will have, and when you should contact him or her with problems. For this prescription to be effective, you should follow your doctor's instructions to the letter. Ask lots of questions and let him or her know what you feel you're capable of doing regarding a decrease in activity. And report back to your doctor about whether you feel your bed rest is helping.

Kinds of Activity Reduction

Because there are many causes and conditions of preterm labor and other complications in pregnancy that are treated with bed rest, no one prescription fits all. Depending on the diagnosis, your doctor may ask you to begin with a relatively modest increase in rest throughout the day to see if this is effective. Or your doctor may start you off on complete bed rest until your contractions or cervical dilation has slowed. Then, if there are no more signs of preterm labor, you may be allowed to slowly increase your level of activity.

The degree of activity reduction ranges from minimal (lying down for an extra hour or two each day, with no heavy lifting or frequent stair climbing) to complete bed rest (lying in bed and being allowed up only to use the bathroom).

If contractions and other signs of preterm labor persist at the activity level you are currently prescribed, your doctor may decide to decrease your level of activity and may prescribe a medication to help stop your contractions, if he or she hasn't already. In some situations the doctor might ask you to lie in a Trendelenberg position, elevating the foot of the bed higher than your head to allow the baby and fluid to completely move away from the cervix. This is done primarily in the hospital if your amniotic membranes appear to be moving out of the cervix and into your vagina.

Degrees of Activity Reduction or Bed Rest

There are four levels or degrees of bed rest. You'll have specific instructions from your doctor about which activities, within the degree of bed rest you are allowed, to continue.

- *Minor Activity Reduction.* This isn't bed rest per se but a request to decrease work hours, or increase rest, particularly if your work requires you to be on your feet a great deal. What your doctor is asking you to do is limit the amount of time you're on your feet. Standing appears to be more harmful than walking, and stair climbing seems to be the most harmful of all because all the abdominal muscles are used.

  If you're an office worker who sits about 80 to 90 percent of the time, increased rest means taking more frequent breaks to take in more fluids, emptying your bladder regularly, and perhaps elevating your feet under your desk with a box or trash can. It also means taking about 10 to 15 minutes to put your feet up and rest when you first get home from work.

  If you have an occupation that requires you to be on your feet more, such as that of nurse or teacher, decreased work hours means taking frequent breaks sitting down with your feet up. It is also important to have a 30 minute rest when you first get home from work, and to make sure you are well hydrated.

Whether you're primarily on your feet or seated at a desk during your workday, decreasing work hours also means you should not be working longer than eight hours a day, jogging, lifting weights, or carrying children.

- *Moderate activity reduction* means further reducing the number and intensity of your activities throughout the day. You'll be encouraged to decrease the number of hours you work by a third if possible. A nap or rest with your feet up for 30 minutes to one hour a day is recommended. The most effective time for resting is when you get home from work, and you should have something to drink before you settle down to rest. Longer rest on your days off is a good idea. If you take care of small children during the day, you should not lift any child weighing over 10 pounds, carry heavy laundry, or climb stairs frequently.

- *Moderate or modified bed rest* is sometimes called "house arrest." This degree of bed rest asks you to stay off your feet most of your day, in bed or on the couch, with your legs off the floor. You should not climb stairs. You're allowed up for a short while to eat meals at the table, make a quick sandwich, or get something to eat or drink. You can also work from the bed or couch if you're doing paperwork, reading, or working on a computer. You will need someone to help you with housekeeping, main meal preparation, transportation, and child care.

- *Strict or complete bed rest* means you're allowed up only to shower, change clothes, go to the bathroom, and go to doctor's appointments. With some physicians strict bed rest means you must also use a bedside commode to go to the bathroom.

Keep in mind, these are general descriptions. There are no strict delineations between the four degrees of bed rest. Check with your doctor about his or her definition of the categories above. Ask for specifics about do's and don'ts. Your doctor's definitions may differ from the ones described above. The following checklist may help both you and your doctor determine what activities will be most therapeutic for maintaining your pregnancy. He or she will probably know what is the most therapeutic for you.

Activity Checklist

The following checklist will help you and your doctor decide exactly what you can and cannot do under your prescription for bed rest. You may want to mark these in pencil rather than pen, or photocopy the pages and take them to your doctor's appointment, because your restrictions may change over the weeks you remain on bed rest.

Activity Guide and Questionnaire for You and Your OB Provider

Instructions: Part A is to be completed by you. Your doctor or midwife will complete Part B, which will give you clear instructions on what activity level to be following. Remember, this will change if your medical situation changes.

PART A: QUESTIONNAIRE FOR THE MOTHER

Name:_____

Birth Date:_____

Doctor/Midwife:_____

Due Date:_____

Occupation:_____

Hours worked per day:_____

Number of small children less than four years of age at your home:_____

Total hours standing at work:_____

Total hours sitting at work:_____

For each question please circle one answer, yes or no.

1. Does work require heavy lifting of any kind?   YES   NO

2. Does work require stair climbing of any kind?   YES   NO

3. Does work require operating heavy machinery of   YES   NO
   any kind?

4. Does work require you to be outside for the   YES   NO
   majority of the day?

5. How many levels (floors) are there in your
   house? _____ Is there a bathroom on every level?   YES   NO

6. Do you have someone who can help with   YES   NO
   housework, meal preparation, grocery shopping,
   transportation, and child care?
   Comments:_____

7. How many hours per day can someone assist you?_____

PART B: ACTIVITY CHECKLIST COMPLETED BY THE OB PROVIDER

OB provider: Please check only one selection per category and indicate
how long this activity is valid (for example, up to the next office visit).

1. Activity Level
No Restrictions _____

Minor Activity Reductions
Frequent breaks at work to take in extra fluids, especially water

_____

No physical or strenuous exercise and no heavy lifting _____

Decrease work hours to _____/day or _____/week

Moderate Activity Reductions
Decrease work hours to _____/day or _____/week

Frequent breaks at work to take in extra fluids, especially water
_____

Increase rest periods _____

No heavy lifting (including children over 10 lbs.) or standing for prolonged time _____

Elevate feet and rest 15 to 30 minutes/day _____

Moderate Bed Rest

Stay off your feet most of your day _____

No stair-climbing _____

Up for a short while for meals or to get something to eat or drink
_____

Frequent intake of extra fluids, especially water _____

Work from the bed or couch, such as paperwork, reading, or working on a computer _____

No going to work, to a gym, or out shopping _____

Need someone to help you with housekeeping, main meal preparation, transportation, and child care _____

Strict Bed Rest
(Same restrictions as moderate bed rest but also including the following)

Allowed up only to shower, go to bathroom, doctor's visits _____

Stop work completely because of_____

Working (including working from home)

Continue working full time_____

Can work part time, number of hours _____

Work at home _____number of hours _____/day or _____/week

Stop work completely because of_____

2. Housework
No restrictions _____

Light housework with no heavy lifting_____

Light housework with no heavy lifting or stair-climbing_____

No housework at all _____

3. Child Care
No restrictions with child care _____

No lifting children _____

Get help with child care at least three hours per day _____

Get help with child care eight hours per day _____

4. Driving
No restrictions _____

Drive only to and from work _____

Drive only to your medical appointment _____

No driving at all _____

5. Sexual Relations
No restrictions _____

Everything permitted except intercourse _____

6. Other Instructions
_____

7. Recommended Consultations
Perinatologist _____

Physical therapist _____

Occupational therapist _____

Neonatologist _____

Social worker _____

Other _____

Adjusting Your Working Life

If you're given a prescription for bed rest, you'll need to inform your employer that you need to alter your work schedule or stop working altogether. This change in your pregnancy and your ability to work can be stressful for you and your family. After all, work is an important part of our lives. Of course, it provides income for our families, but it also gives us a sense of accomplishment.

You may have an occupation that allows you some flexibility with your work responsibilities or schedule. You should talk to your employer to see if you can temporarily switch to another job that does not require a lot of physical or mental stress.

Another option is to check with your employer to see if you can do some or most of your work from home. You'll also need to discuss this solution with your doctor or midwife. You will probably not be able to maintain the schedule you normally have when you're actually at the office, and you should communicate your limitations to your employer. Sometimes you can do your job partially or keep working from your bed until certain projects are done.

Keep in mind that the point of reducing your activity or of bed rest is to give your body a chance to rest by easing up on stress in your life and to see if your condition improves. The paramount goal is to give your baby every opportunity to get to full term and be born healthy.

If you cannot do your job anywhere but your worksite:

- Discuss your options with your employer; see if you can transfer to a job temporarily that will allow you to work from home.
- Check with your employer to see if you are eligible to apply for either sick leave or disability or both. If so, take forms to your OB provider to sign.

- Check whether your employer will allow donations of sick leave from coworkers, to avoid using all your leave or be off work without pay.
- Check with your benefit administrator at work to see if you have a separate disability insurance coverage, and if you do, activate it.
- Prepare for extra costs. Disability payments are usually a percentage of your income. There may be unexpected costs for child care, extra medical costs not covered by insurance, and costs for housecleaning and takeout dinners if your partner can't manage these additional duties on top of his job.
- Know that you are entitled to some job protection. Current federal law requires employers to abide by the Family Leave Act, which allows full-time employees 12 weeks of unpaid emergency leave each year.
- Check your local Social Services department to find out about local and national financial assistance if your income drops significantly due to complications in your pregnancy that need to be treated with bed rest. Ask specifically about the food supplement program for pregnant women called Women Infant and Children (WIC).

Keep in mind that being on bed rest is only temporary! The purpose is to get your baby to a healthy birth. Your partner can help with the housework. Your friends and family can help with the other children, but *only you can grow this baby inside your body.*

Managing Your Space

Even if you're not on bed rest, but you're told you need to decrease your workload and get more rest, it's important to arrange your home to decrease your activity level. You want to find a place or several places where you can rest even if they require that your partner to do minor rearranging of furniture or cleaning to prepare these areas for you. Even for bed rest, you do not necessarily need to be in bed, in the bedroom, the entire time, which can be very boring and isolating. Try setting up two areas, one in the bedroom for sleeping and alone time,

TRY THIS

- Review your bed rest activity list.
- Make a "To Do" list of all the things you're responsible for on a weekly to monthly basis.
- Include all the items that may need to be eliminated to decrease your stress, such as bill paying, grocery shopping, child care, elder parent care, pet care, and volunteer work, etc.
- List all the people in your life whom you can ask for help. Leave no one out: family in and out of the area, neighbors, friends, coworkers, church groups, volunteer groups, babysitters, organizations, etc.
- Match the helpers with the tasks. Ask your partner for help if doing this task is stressful. You'll be surprised that many people, including strangers, are more than willing to help.

and another in a communal area where the rest of the family can visit with you and help you feel you are in touch with the world.

Here are some suggestions to make your space comfortable:

- Place your main rest area near a window, to take advantage of natural light. This will keep you from getting claustrophobic and the light will help improve your mood.
- Have a portable reading light that can move with you.
- Have your main resting area near a bathroom.
- Get pillows and more pillows. A bed quickly becomes unbearable if there's no way to alter its contours. There are specially made pillows designed for bed resters, but any assortment of pillows—hard, soft, small, big, or long pillow rolls—will help create new positions. You may also want to put an egg crate mattress pad on the sofa or bed to soften the surface without losing firmness.
- Have a portable telephone or cell phone and important phone numbers easily accessible, including the telephone book. Remember that although cordless phones and cell phones are conven-

ient, they do need to be recharged. Choose a place where cradle and handset can be within easy reach.

- Keep nearby a backpack filled with your personal address book, watch, date book, writing pads, pens, and a portable writing surface like a clipboard with a pen tied to it or a lap-pad, that is a flat board with a squishy pillow attached to the underside. These will help you to write in a prone position. If you have a pen attached to the writing surface, you won't need to get up if your last pen rolls off the bedside table and under the bed. The backpack will be helpful to transport items when you need to move to another room.

- Keep this book, your pregnancy notebook, and other reference books in arm's reach. Write down questions for your doctor and anything you think might be important information.

- Keep with you a journal to write down what's happening to you and your pregnancy and your feelings about it. You may also want to write about the events of each day, such as visits from friends. Many mental health professionals say people handle their situations better if they can document their thoughts in a journal. This journal will be a record of your extraordinary efforts on behalf of your baby.

- Having books, magazines, catalogs, your hobby (like needlework) or an activity for the day, radio or tape player, calendar, clock, and even a laptop computer will probably fill more than your bedside table. Laundry baskets or sturdy shopping bags are helpful for sorting supplies and can be easily moved when needed. Do not lift them yourself if they are heavy.

- Have a TV, radio, electronic video games, DVD player, or VCR nearby to help keep you up to date on news and offer some entertainment. Have healthy snacks and plenty of water within your reach, without having to get out of bed. If you're going to be alone all day, a cooler filled with complete meals should also be placed near your area.

- Rent or buy a table like they have in hospitals, which extends over the bed, forming a surface for writing, eating, and other activities that need a flat, firm surface. These tables are usually on wheels. Any kind of rolling table is helpful because it can be moved easily and you can push it aside when it's not needed. Some experienced bed resters use a sturdy ironing board or light computer table.

- Have a basket of toys, puzzles, or books that you can share with your children. Allow them some personal time in bed with you for cuddling and visiting.
- You may also find a "grabber" or "snatcher" helpful. By squeezing the handle, this sticklike device can retrieve smaller objects that are out of arm's reach.
- Keep your medications, in a plastic bag with a small note pad to keep track of when you last took any medications and when they need to be refilled.
- Put old sheets on your bed and couch. They're usually softer and comfortable, and you won't mind if they get soiled or stained.
- Keep your lotions, lip balm, hairbrush, mirror, and makeup nearby, in case someone surprises you with a visit. You may feel better knowing you can fix your appearance quickly and easily.
- Tape emergency or important phone numbers on the phone or on your table. Include in this list your doctor/midwife's office, the hospital, your partner's number, the day care/babysitter, and a reliable friend or neighbor's contact information.

Be the Director, Not an Actor

It is very hard to do bed rest alone. The chores you can no longer do may have to be done by your partner, but ask family and friends to pitch in as well. *Do not be shy*. Ask for what you want and need. Direct others to how they can help, in fact make a list of things you and your partner need help with and ask family members and friends to choose one. It helps to be specific. Make the grocery list, naming the preferred brands. If you have a supportive group, ask them to organize a rotation of visits, home-cooked meals, and other activities that will support you and lighten your partner's burden.

Many friends initially can't understand how having to stay in bed or on the sofa all day can be that bad. Or some can't understand why you can't just take a break from the bed rest and join them with on an outing or activity. Ask them to come visit to help pass the time if you are feeling up to it. If these friends are very close, you may want to communicate your worries about the baby and your partner, who may be floundering under the added responsibility and his or her own worries. Another sympathetic and resourceful ear is a support group for women on bed rest. You will need a circle of supportive people for emotional as well as practical support. Find out the best time to call friends and family who can be counted on to listen sympathetically or provide you with diversion in the form of humor and stories. If you start to feel guilty about taking up their time, remember that they realize that however much work they're doing on your behalf, your job is the hardest of all.

Your Personal Challenge

Even though you're confined to bed or home for a serious medical condition, you'll look fine to others; in fact, you may look terrific with all the extra rest. You won't seem sick, and for most of you, you won't feel sick. Many people around you will think you can do many of the activities you did before because they see no outward change in you. You'll have to educate them that what you're doing is not by choice but a necessary prescription from your doctor to help your baby have enough time to grow and be healthy.

> **KEY THOUGHT TO REMEMBER**
> You may struggle with the thought that during the bed rest period, you don't have a bandage, cast, or sickly pallor to explain even to yourself, your being off work, at home, and doing "nothing."

Although some may have difficulty sympathizing with your plight, the person who will struggle the most with your activity restrictions will probably be you. Your most important challenge is to understand and accept these restrictions and agree to maintain them.

Typically, you'll probably feel tired at first, grateful for the chance to rest. After a few days of rest you may feel energetic. All too quickly, however, you may feel anxious, and then bored. You'll find yourself justifying why you can get up and out of bed and even run errands. It will start with you staying up longer than usual, or just doing a tiny amount of straightening up. Then you'll find yourself making excuses for a quick trip out of your home. Or you may get up to go to the bathroom, notice that there are towels on the floor or the sink, or that the tub needs cleaning, and before you realize it, you're actually cleaning the bathroom.

You need to see yourself as someone who has a cast on each leg. If you were hobbled, you would never dream of driving a car or climbing stairs or loading the dishwasher, would you? Tell yourself: The more you do that is not permitted, the guiltier you'll feel—especially if you find yourself on the way to the hospital or doctor's office with increased contractions. And remind yourself that increased guilt will only increase your stress. By the same token, forgive yourself if you do break the rules and promise yourself to start over again with a stronger commitment.

Using Signals

Again, bed rest can be very hard to accept and endure. It's not as easy as it might seem to others. On a regular basis, describe your feelings and frustrations to your partner or a good friend. Decide together on a nonverbal signal that person can give you when he or she feels you're doing too much; nonverbal, because a verbal signal risks hurting your feelings. Perhaps your partner could plump up a certain pillow to signal that you're more active than you should be. Agree beforehand that this is only a signal and you won't argue about it; you can choose to accept the signal or ignore it. However, remember that the physician has put you in charge of following his or her directions and your partner in charge of supporting you.

You can establish another nonverbal signal to let your partner or friend know you need more support to endure the bed rest and you feel you're going crazy because of it. Write him or her a little note about what you are missing or craving. Perhaps you're desperate for a vacation. Together, plan ways to get you back on track. You might try changing your environment to another room, watching travel or previous vacation videos, having a picnic on the floor, lying on a lounge chair on the patio and having a cookout, or having a movie night with a video, popcorn, drinks, and cuddling on the couch together.

Bed Rest and Depression

It's important to be aware of the signs of depression, so you can ask for help if you feel you're experiencing the blues for extended periods. Bed rest shakes the optimism of even the emotionally sunniest. A health care professional should have the opportunity to determine if your blues warrant counseling, or whether antidepressants are required to help you through your pregnancy and bed rest.

> **KEY THOUGHT TO REMEMBER**
> Every day on bed rest is a gift you're giving your baby that could affect the rest of his or her life.

Even if you don't feel that you're clinically depressed, you may have difficulty keeping up your morale. Take one day at a time. Think of yourself as living each moment to help your baby. Write a letter to your baby describing what you're feeling and how much you love him or her. Write about who you are and who you will be in his or her life. Next, write a letter to yourself about how things are going and how you hope to make it through this difficult time. Open these letters when you feel the most frustrated with bed rest.

Keeping Control of Your Time

Feeling satisfaction at accomplishing things is very important to everyone's mental health. Successful bed resters have found that creating a schedule for your days will help you manage your time and make you feel more productive. And conversely, feeling that you're not getting anything done—even though helping your baby is getting something very important done—may lead you to blues and depression.

You may not be in charge of the fact that you are having a complication that requires you to stay in bed, but you really are in charge of what you make of this situation, and you can turn it into a productive time. And you'll feel better if you're busy because it will help pass the time.

Get an appointment book with the days broken down by hours. Create a schedule for what you want to accomplish each day. Start with your daily wake-up time. Fill in your meal times and your time with children and spouse. Then write in other routine tasks such as a shower, hair care, and so on. Include times for work if you'll be working during bed rest. Schedule time for things you enjoy doing like reading or hobbies. Try to alternate tasks that use your brain and your body. You can even include deadlines if it challenges you to complete tasks. Review this daily schedule each morning and amend it to include unexpected but welcome visits from your mother or a friend, or a trip out of the house to the doctor's.

Here's a sample to give you some idea of what to include in your own schedule:

Time	Suggested Activity Options	Sample Schedule
6:30 am	Wake up/bathroom.	Wake up/bathroom
7:00 am	Breakfast with partner/ review day and provide partner with list of shopping.	Breakfast with partner
7:30 am	Get family off to work or school. Meditate, relaxation techniques, journal writing, review the calendar.	Meditate, relaxation techniques
8:00 am	Read the newspaper or listen to the news (brain).	Read the newspaper
8:30–9:00	Bed exercises and stretches (body).	Exercises and stretches (body)
9:30–10:30	Read novel, make a grocery list, write a letter, type on the computer or search the Internet, go catalog shopping (brain).	Search the Internet
10:30–12:00 noon	Listen to music, but sing the words and move your arms to the rhythm, practice a foreign language out loud, call a friend or catch up with colleagues at work, match socks or fold towels sitting down (body).	Listen to music and sing the words and move your arms to the rhythm

12:00 noon–12:30 p.m.	LUNCH. Set up your area. Concentrate on your food. Before eating, observe the color, feel the texture, savor the aroma, then taste each item. You'll enjoy your meal more with this conscious effort.	LUNCH—set up your area
12:30–1:00	Straighten your area, put away your eating utensils, wash your face and hands, put on makeup and fix your hair. Do your nails or massage your arms and legs with moisturizers (body).	Wash your face and hands, put on makeup
1:00–1:30	Research your pregnancy condition, calls to organizations, check on support lines for women on bed rest. Read your books on pregnancy, breastfeeding, or child care (brain).	Check on support lines for women on bed rest
1:30–2:30	Listen to soft music or take a nap.	Listen to soft music or take a nap
2:30–4:30	Work on project such as knitting, making new address book, a scrapbook or filling a photo album, organizing bills. Write out thank-you notes, make a list of baby items you still need to buy. (Brain.)	Write out thank-you notes, make a list of baby items you still need to buy
4:30–6:00	Watch a movie or listen to a book on tape.	Watch a movie
6:00–6:30	Straighten your area, do some exercise, decide what you want to do with your partner tonight—watch TV, play cards, have friends over, etc) (Body.)	Do some exercise
6:30–7:30	DINNER with partner, review the day, what you've learned, what you've accomplished.	DINNER with partner
7:30–Bedtime	Watch TV, play cards, have friends over, etc.	Have friends over

Remember, you're in charge! Keep in mind that this schedule is for you. If you find that you don't want to do the selected thing in the time slot, shorten the time allotted or switch it to another time slot. And conversely, if you find you're engrossed in your novel and want to keep reading beyond the hour allotted, by all means, do so.

Engage in Projects

Don't be surprised if you don't enjoy doing things you did prior to being on bed rest. It's just a reaction to the change in your circumstances, the physical demands of pregnancy, and the fatigue of bed rest. Think about several projects you've always meant to do if you just had some extra time. We say *several* because if you decide to just read novels for the next six weeks, you'll probably quickly decide that reading is the last thing you feel like doing. Here are some suggestions:

- Make a new address book—consolidating from all your older ones. Call your relatives and friends to confirm that their numbers and street addresses are accurate. This gives you a chance to let them know what's happening to you and to get support from them.
- Learn a language using tapes. Most people don't have the time in their daily lives to practice learning a new language. This project is also easy to do lying down.
- Learn to knit or crochet. Ask a friend who knows how to start you off on a simple item.
- Start reading books that have sounded interesting to you but you just never got around to. Make a list of books your partner or a friend can get from the local library or bookstore.
- Watch television. You may want to tape your favorite shows so you can watch them at different times or be able to shut them off if someone comes to visit.
- Rent tapes or DVDs from that long list of films you've always wanted to see.
- Look into childbirth education classes if you haven't had a chance to take them or complete them. Many instructors will

give private lessons in your home for you and your partner or can refer you to someone who offers this service. Your part-ner can tour the hospital labor and delivery rooms and bring back photos or videotape the tour. Your childbirth educator may also know how to contact other couples going through bed rest.

- Get contact information from your doctor or midwife about other couples going through your situation, or better yet, about a couple who has successfully gone through a bed rest pregnancy. Many women use the Internet to communicate with other moth-ers on bed rest.
- Learn everything you can about your condition, the condition of your baby, and what to expect if, despite the bed rest, your baby has to be delivered early.
- Ask your family and friends about things they would like to do if they had the time. You may even be able to earn a little money by doing these projects for them. Ideas include offer-ing to make a new address book for them, addressing wedding invitations—if you have nice handwriting and can do this in a prone position—or doing some research by telephone or Internet.
- Volunteer to record yourself reading a book out loud for the blind, or check with a local volunteer bank about stuffing envelopes for your favorite charity.
- With doctor approval, do the stretches and exercises described in the next section.

Stretches and Exercises

Note: Make sure you get permission from your doctor for doing any stretching and very light exercising while on bed rest.

With the above caution in mind, we suggest you do the following stretches and exercises regularly each day. In addition, if you can afford them and it's okay with your doctor, massages from a massage thera-pist who comes to your home may be helpful to ease sore body parts and for a general sense of well-being.

Staying in Tone, Keeping Muscles in Shape

Plan some part of your day for doing the following exercises. In preparation, follow the recommendations below.

1. Have a light meal about an hour before you exercise.
2. Empty your bladder.
3. Wear loose clothing.
4. Keep water nearby.
5. Choose music you like.
6. Watch your level of exertion; it should always feel easy, never arduous.
7. Stop exercising if you feel out of breath, contractions, or any other discomfort.
8. Experiment with different times of day, to find when you enjoy exercising the most.
9. Give yourself a massage by gently rubbing, your arms, legs, feet, hands, neck, temples, shoulders, and back to warm the muscles.

Muscle Toning Exercises

1. Sitting cross-legged, lift your shoulders toward your ears and roll them around to the back and down to a relaxed-shoulders dropped position. Do a set of eight. (You can increase the number of sets, as you feel able.) These are shoulder rolls.
2. Sitting cross-legged with your arms relaxed, lift and lower your forearms in sets of eight. These are biceps curls.
3. Sitting cross-legged, reach overhead as if you're reaching for a rope dangling from above. Alternate the arm that is reaching for the rope. This is called rope climbing.
4. Lying on your left side, draw your knees toward your chest to round the lower back while you exhale. When you inhale, relax your knees and let them drop farther away from your chest. These are pelvic rocks.
5. Lying on your left side, make your body into the shape of a chair. Lift your upper leg without twisting in the hip. Hold a second and lower. Do a set of eight, then repeat the exercise while lying on your right side. These are bent leg lifts.

6. In any position, consciously tell your body to pull in the muscles around your vulva and vagina. It may feel like you're trying to hold urine in. Hold a few seconds and release. These are Kegel exercises.
7. Kneeling on all fours, round your back up toward the ceiling like a cat arching its back. Hold for a few seconds and release while exhaling. Do several times.

Stretching Exercises
1. Sitting cross-legged and facing forward, tilt your head toward your right shoulder and hold for about eight seconds, breathing normally. Repeat on the left side.
2. In any relaxed position, squeeze you eyes shut and then open them wide. Keep your eyes open and, without moving your head, look to the far right and then slowly to the left. Repeat with wide-open eyes, looking up and then down. Close your eyes and breathe, and rest for a minute.
3. Sitting cross-legged, wrap your arms around your shoulders as if giving yourself a hug. Hold for eight seconds and release. Repeat several times.
4. Lying on your left side with your knees bent, lift your upper leg from beneath the thigh and gently pull your thigh toward your chest. Do not press hard on the baby. Do several repetitions and repeat the exercise while lying on your right side.
5. Lying on your left side, lift your upper leg a little and flex your toes back toward you. Return your leg to atop the other leg. Do not point your foot, since this may cause cramps. Repeat several times and repeat the exercise while lying on your right side.

Your Children

If you have other children, you'll need to make arrangements for child care in your home or with a babysitter. There should always be another adult in the home if you're on bed rest and your children are less than six years old.

If you've been the primary care giver for your child or children until you were put on bed rest, there will probably be a period of adjustment for everyone. You may find it easier to send the children to a sitter each day so you can truly rest, because you may be inclined to submit to helping him or her out as part of your mothering routine. The sitter will also be a good option if you have to leave your home suddenly if you're having medical problems. Or you may find it less stressful to have your children with you at home, but with a very perceptive babysitter who can engage your child with activities in another area allowing you to rest.

You may be able to count on family members for your babysitting needs. It's easier on everyone when the children are familiar with their care givers, but this may not be feasible because of the amount of babysitting time required. Regardless of outside or in-home child care, make a conscious effort to spend an hour or so with your children every day.

Here are some things you can do with your children while you're on bed rest:

- Plan craft activities they can do on your bed using your writing board.
- Select a chapter book and read one or two chapters to them each day.
- Have snack or "tea" time with them and find out how their day has gone.
- Pick out their clothes together and do their hair.
- Spend time helping them with homework.
- Plan a birthday party or some special activity for after the baby is born.
- Explain to them that lying in bed is helping their brother or sister get bigger. Let them hear the baby's heartbeat and feel for kicks. Solicit their help by asking them to get you things in other parts of the house. This will empower them. Avoid telling them about the things that may go wrong with your pregnancy as this may be too scary for them.

Activities with a Toddler

You may not be able to arrange full-time child care while you're on bed rest. If you find yourself alone with your toddler for a short time, how can you stick to your bed rest restrictions and keep an active toddler happy?

Here are some suggestions from mothers who were on bed rest with a toddler:

- If it's possible, set up your toddler's favorite activities in your room, like a train set or doll house.
- Move yourself to the play area and recline on a mattress on the floor.
- Keep diaper supplies nearby or feed your toddler in a car seat next to your rest area.
- Have someone prepare a box of activities. Items in the box may include coloring and sticker books, paper, scissors, glue sticks, crayons, books, and puzzles.
- Create make-believe activities. For instance, if you both like going to the zoo, make your own zoo with his or her stuffed animals. Have your child place the animals around the room and make a visit to each and tell you what it's doing. You can expand on this activity by reading books and watching videos about animals. Or pretend with your toddler that he or she is a baby animal being born, given a name, and fed for the first time.
- If you both like music, put on a tape and have your child sing and dance or play an instrument.
- When all else fails, there are always children's videos.
- Try napping while your child does.
- Remember that your priority is the child inside you. If you feel tempted to get up with your toddler, remind yourself you would not get up if you had two broken legs!

What should you tell your toddler about your situation? Some women explain that mommy has to stay in bed to help the baby grow. They plant seeds in cups or small pots with their children as a long-term project to mark the passage of the days or you can make a paper chain for each week you need to be on bedrest, and pull one link off each Monday. You can also mark the days together on a calendar and fill in each space with stickers and drawings that illustrate what has happened each day.

Bed Rest and Your Partner

When you're put on bed rest, your partner will be precipitously thrust into multiple roles. He may have no previous experience with many of these roles. Suddenly, he'll have to create a safe and comfortable environment in the home for you, keep the home clean and stocked with nourishing and tasty food, pick up and retrieve other children from day care or school, perhaps communicate your condition and give updates to family members and friends, and continue to attend to his or her full-time job. On top of these duties, he'll no doubt be reacting to your state of mind about this turn of events and have worries about your health and the health of the baby. Your partner will need support!

He may not be able to articulate his feelings and needs, or may be reticent about "complaining" at all when you're the one who's going through the discomforts of bed rest. He may also feel lonely because the attention he's accustomed to getting from you is not available.

You can look for ways to show that you appreciate all that he's trying to do. Try not to complain about less than pristine surroundings, the formerly white underwear that's now pink, and strangely cooked meals. Find ways to talk with your partner about how he's feeling, and encourage him to seek out and spend time with other men in the same situation. Remind him of the wonderful times you will have together in the near future.

Managing Bed Rest

We hope this chapter has alleviated some of your concerns about bed rest and that you've found suggestions on how to manage its challenges. These suggestions were taken from our pregnancies, some of which included bed rest, and from interviews with other women on bed rest. We hope a few of the ideas included in this chapter will help you survive activity reduction during your pregnancy.

10

Carrying Twins or More

 Rachel's Journal

> *Dear Journal,*
>   *I met Becky and her two-year-old twin boys today. I'm so glad Dr. Wells suggested I get to know some moms with twins. She made it look pretty easy. I'm actually excited to be having two at once. Just three months to go!*

Many people are caught off guard with the news that they are going to have twins. You and your partner may be dumbfounded, then exhilarated, and then anxious when you first hear you're having twins or more. You may dwell on fears about how taxing it will be to care for more than one baby. On the other hand, if you've been trying to get pregnant for some time, part of you is very excited that you've achieved your goal.

All of these reactions are common and normal. While you may be focusing on the outcome of your pregnancy—your babies and your life thereafter—your doctor will be focusing on your immediate pregnancy and your babies while in the uterus. A pregnancy with multiples is considered high-risk. You will have special care throughout the nine months.

If you haven't been pregnant or given birth before, all the changes and physical complaints of a pregnancy with multiples will seem as they should be, and not unusual in your eyes. After all, you won't have personal experience to draw from and you won't know what to expect. However, if you've had other children, you may find yourself comparing this special pregnancy to what you experienced in the past.

KAREN AND SCOTT'S STORY

Karen and Scott walked into the hospital radiology unit holding hands. Each knew what the other was thinking. Something must be wrong with their baby. Why else would Dr. Davis have asked Karen to get a sonogram as soon as possible?

A nurse called from a doorway, and they followed her into a darkened room. Karen lay back on the exam table and pulled up her shirt, exposing her newly swelling abdomen. The radiologist, Dr. Powell, entered the room and shook both Karen's and Scott's hands.

"Have you ever had a sonogram, Karen?" Dr. Powell asked.

Karen shook her head no and watched as the doctor shook a plastic bottle and squirted some warmed, jellylike substance onto her abdomen. Then he rolled the transducer through the jelly, causing gray, black, and white fuzzy objects to appear on a TV screen.

"We don't usually feel the need to do sonograms on someone as early in pregnancy as you are," he said, "but Dr. Davis thought he could hear . . . " Dr. Powell's voice drifted off as he made a few maneuvers across Karen's slippery stomach. Then he stopped moving and pushed a button to freeze the image.

"Well, there you are!" Dr. Powell exclaimed.

Karen and Scott could see nothing but blobs. "What is it?" Scott whispered.

"Well, the 'it' is a 'they'!" the doctor said. "You're going to have twins. There are two babies in there."

"Twins!" Scott gulped.

"Dr. Davis thought he could hear two heartbeats, but he wanted to be sure." Dr. Powell continued as his free hand traced the outline of two bodies on the TV screen.

"Twins?" Karen said, finally finding her voice.

The doctor slid the transducer across her stomach a few more times and brought the babies into view from another angle

"Their size is right where they should be for your dates. They're only about two inches long now. Each will grow to the size of a normal baby by the time you're ready to deliver. I'm afraid *you* will get enormous, however," Dr. Powell said teasingly.

Karen grinned in mock horror and went back to looking for her babies on the screen. Scott was still trying to make sense of this new development. "Twins! But there are no twins in either of our families."

Dr. Powell asked them to make an appointment with Dr. Davis and said he would relay the sonogram information to the office. To be continued . . .

It may be difficult at times. At times, you may feel overwhelmed by the discomfort of carrying two or more babies, or you may have a great deal of anxiety about the outcome. Try to surround yourself with supportive family and friends and health care professionals who can help. Try to find other couples who have had twins or more who can "show you the ropes." You may need these support contacts for suggestions on how to cope with the actual problems or merely feel reassured by spending time with couples who've been through a pregnancy with twins or more. Many people want to help you. There's no need to tough it out alone.

Signs of a Multiple (Gestation) Pregnancy

With current technology, diagnosing a multiple pregnancy can occur earlier than was possible in the past. A multiple pregnancy may be discovered in several ways:

- During an ultrasound, your doctor or a technician can see more than one baby. Today, most multiple births are discovered in this way.
- The measurement of your uterus is larger than usual for the number of weeks you have been pregnant. OB providers refer to this circumstance as "size greater than dates." Your predicted *fundal height*—the measurement from your pubic bone to the top of the uterus, or the *fundus*—is greater than it should be. If your measurements are larger than expected, you may be having a large baby or you may be carrying more than one baby.
- Your doctor or midwife, using a Doppler or fetoscope, hears more than one fetal heartbeat. It is very difficult to detect two or more distinct and different heartbeats. Prior to the use of

ultrasound, detecting more than one heartbeat was the only method available. As you can imagine, many multiples went undetected.

- The results of an *alpha fetoprotein* (AFP) *screen* or *triple screen* are abnormal. Results from this routine prenatal screening test for neural tube defect are based on a presumed singleton pregnancy, your age, and the number of weeks into the pregnancy. If you're carrying undiagnosed multiples, the test results are usually abnormal. This requires that you undergo additional evaluation, including an advanced ultrasound that can confirm your pregnancy with multiples.

Pregnant with Twins, or Even More

Perhaps your doctor has just announced that you're pregnant with twins, or with triplets, quadruplets, or even quintuplets. Or perhaps you're about to undergo fertility treatments and you know you're at an increased risk for having a multiple pregnancy. You may have heard the scary words "high-risk pregnancy" and want to know what this means for you. Well, increasingly, you are not alone. Having multiples is becoming more common. According to the Center for Disease Control:

- From 1980 to 1997 the number of sets of twins born doubled (from 68,339 to 104,137).
- In the same period, the number of triplets and higher-order multiples quadrupled (from 1337 to 6737).[1]

This phenomenal rise in the number of multiples is attributed to two changes in birthing patterns in the last two decades:

1. More women are having babies later in their lives than in previous decades. As a woman ages, she becomes more likely to release more than one egg at ovulation, and therefore has more of a chance that more than one egg will be fertilized and possibly result in twins, triplets, or more.
2. More women have fertility treatments available to them especially when nowadays some states mandate benefits for fertility

services. Sometimes these treatments result in more that one fertilized egg, and thus more than one baby.

One-third of the rise in the number of multiples born is attributed to older age at pregnancy and two-thirds to the use of fertility treatments. Most twins (71 percent) are still being born to younger mothers, those 25 to 39 years old. But most of the *increase* in the number of twins has come from women over 30, and especially women over 40. There has been a 63 percent increase in women 40 to 44 having twins, and *a 1000 percent increase* among women over the ages of 45 to 49.[2] Again, as noted above, most of these women have used assisted reproductive technology to achieve their pregnancies.

Twins are not the only result of fertility treatments. Triplets, quadruplets, quintuplets, sextuplets, and septuplets have also increased in number. In the last decade, these "higher-order" multiples have increased 400 percent for women over 30 and 1000 percent for women over 40.[3]

Fraternal and Identical Twins

Twins are unique among multiples in that a third of them are identical. To explain this, you must know that there are two ways a twin pregnancy can occur.

Identical twins occur when one fertilized egg splits into two embryos sometime in the first 10 days after conception. Identical twins are also referred to as *monozygotic*, which means one zygote, or one egg. Fraternal twins, which are three times as common as identical twins, occur when two eggs are fertilized.

Identical twins have the same genetic makeup, or genes, which means they have the same physical characteristics, hair color, and eye color. They are always the same gender and have the same blood type. Multiples from different eggs may be similar in appearance, but they are definitely not identical in genetic makeup. They can have different hair and eye color, be different sexes, and have different blood types. Identical twins occur in only one set out of 250 births.[4]

There can also be fraternal triplets, quadruplets, quintuplets, etc. In these cases, several eggs are fertilized at one time by an equal number of sperm. In very rare instances, a couple of eggs are fertilized but then one of these eggs splits, resulting in a pair of identical babies among fraternal siblings. This situation is most common in triplets.

Another very rare occurrence is the fertilization of eggs at different times. The babies that result are of different gestational ages. An even rarer occurrence is fertilization of eggs at different times and with different sperm from different fathers. This results in multiples that are genetically related only through the mother.

Family History

Identical twins are simply a surprise in nature; no one can predict this type of twinning. However, having fraternal twins can be determined by your genetic history, not your partner's. This means that you have inherited a tendency to release more than one egg at ovulation. It doesn't matter how many sperm your partner produces, the number of eggs determines the number of babies. If you have a family history of twins, you will have a greater chance of having fraternal twins.

The Possibilities

You have an increased chance of having fraternal twins if:

- You've had previous pregnancies.
- You're over 35.
- You've taken fertility medications.
- You're taller or larger than the average woman.
- You conceived in the month that followed stopping hormonal contraception.

To explain this last point: For some time after stopping birth control pills, your body retains an elevated level of the hormone gonadotropin. This hormone can stimulate more than one egg to be released at ovulation. Thus, to avoid a multiple pregnancy, most OB providers usually recommend waiting three months after stopping hormone-based contraception before trying to conceive.

Recent statistics from the Center for Disease Control show that:

- About 30 African-American twins are born per 1000 births.
- About 27 Caucasian twins are born per 1000 births.
- About 19 Hispanic twins are born per 1000 births.[5]

Telling the Difference Between Twin Types

If you're carrying twins, your doctor may use ultrasound to try to determine whether they will be fraternal or identical twins. The doctor looks for several things.

First of all, if ultrasound reveals that the babies are of different sexes, the twins, of course, are fraternal. But keep in mind that ultrasound may not be able to determine the sex of each twin.

Next, your doctor looks at the placentas. Fraternal twins definitely have their own placentas, whereas identical twins may or may not share one placenta. Therefore, having two placentas doesn't rule out identical twins.

Finally, your doctor will look at the membranes surrounding the developing embryos. There are two parts of the membranes. The *chorion* is the outer membrane that surrounds the amniotic sac or sacs. The *amnion*, also referred to as the amniotic sac, is the inner membrane. Most twin pregnancies have two amniotic sacs, but they may have a single chorion. Identifying a single chorion means the twins are identical. It's very difficult using ultrasound alone to determine whether there is only one chorion, and therefore difficult to definitely say that the twins are identical.

Amniocentesis and chromosomal testing of the amniotic fluid is another way to tell whether the twins are identical or fraternal, if you opt to have this test. Often, however, final determination will often have to wait until after the babies are born and their placentas can be examined.

Identical but Different

There are several different kinds of identical twins. How the embryos will develop in the pregnancy is determined by when the fertilized egg separates.

- When the egg separates early in the implantation stage, the twins will each have their own amnion, chorion, and placenta. This is called *diamnionic* and *dichorionic*, meaning there are two amniotic sacs and two chorions.
- If the splitting occurs a little later after fertilization, the twins each have their own amnion but will share a single chorion, and the placentas will join together. Obstetric providers call this situation *diamnionic* and *monochorionic*, meaning two amnions and one chorion.
- If the separation of the fertilized egg occurs even later after fertilization, the twins will share all three parts: amnion, chorion, and placenta. These twins are called *monoamniotic* and *monochorionic*. This type of identical twin set is very rare and can cause more pregnancy complications than the two mentioned above. When identical twins form more than 10 days after fertilization, the twins will be conjoined (will share body parts).

Potential Complications for Monoamniotic and Monochorionic Twins

If you're carrying twins that are in the same sac, there's some danger that their umbilical cords may wrap around each other, constricting oxygen flow. In this case, your pregnancy will be monitored with frequent sonograms and you'll be asked to keep fetal movement records daily. The difficulty of this assignment will be trying to determine which baby is moving.

Another potential complication of monoamniotic/monochorionic twins is the "twin-to-twin transfusion syndrome." Because the blood vessels are so closely situated in one amniotic sac, blood and nutrients can pass through one twin and be sent on to the other, depriving the first of sustenance and keeping it from growing normally. Both babies can have complications from this syndrome.

Having monoamniotic/monochorionic twins is extremely rare. If you're pregnant with this kind of twin pregnancy, your doctor may refer you to a perinatologist, the specialist in high-risk pregnancies, who can perform a number of specialized examinations of the babies.

How Having More than One Is Different There are differences between a singleton pregnancy and a multiple pregnancy. The continuation of Karen and Scott's story will illustrate how a pregnancy with multiples is different than one with one baby. The italicized words and phrases indicate medical care specific to a multiple pregnancy.

KAREN AND SCOTT'S STORY (Continued)

Early Pregnancy with Multiples

Karen and Scott went to see her doctor the same week she was diagnosed with twins, and Dr. Davis explained that she and Scott would have to make a decision about the rest of her care. He told them that even though twin pregnancies are fairly common, she would need to be watched more closely. In his practice, he said, he had successfully managed women carrying twins in *consultation* with two specialists—a perinatologist and a nutritionist. They could opt to continue her prenatal care with him alternating some of her visits with the perinatologist or completely transfer all of her care to a perinatologist. He suggested they meet with a perinatologist to help them decide, and let him know which route they had opted for.

A week later Karen and Scott went to see Dr. Nelson, whose practice included a nutritionist, a sonotechnologist, and a full-time nurse who would be assigned to coordinate Karen's care. After discussing their options with Dr. Nelson, Karen and Scott decided that since her office was near Scott's, and because of her experience with twin pregnancies, they would continue the rest of Karen's care with her.

The next time Karen saw Dr. Nelson, the doctor reviewed her medical history, gave Karen a *vaginal exam, and explained that mothers carrying twins are examined frequently* because of their increased risk of preterm labor and premature delivery. Dr. Nelson gave Karen *a small notebook that described pregnancy with multiples.* It included blank pages, so she could write down information specific to her pregnancy or questions she wanted to remember to ask. Dr. Nelson reiterated that Karen *would have more frequent prenatal visits* than women with singleton pregnancies.

Looking at the calendar, Karen was shocked to see how much time prenatal appointments were going to take out of her work schedule. She made a note to herself to let her supervisor at work know that this change in her pregnancy would require more time off. Dr. Nelson concluded the visit by assuring her that every thing looked good and told her to continue her normal routine.

Next, Karen went to see the nurse in charge of her case, Susan, who gave Karen *her direct telephone number* and encouraged her to *call with questions at any time.* Susan said she would be contacting her at least every other week to check on how she was doing. She encouraged Karen to think about signing up for a childbirth education class that would help prepare her and Scott for labor and delivery. Together, they went over Karen's level of rest and exercise and looked for ways to increase both.

Susan noted that though *rest and exercise* are very important in all pregnancies, they are especially important for women carrying multiples. She suggested Karen take slow walks every day and try doing some exercises to increase strength in her back and arms, since she would eventually be carrying a lot of weight in front. Later in her pregnancy, Susan warned Karen, she would probably need to take time off of work to further increase her rest.

Susan showed Karen the OB practice's *nonstress-test machine, specially designed to monitor two babies' heart rates at the same time.* They also visited the ultrasound room. Kyle, the ultrasound technologist, told Karen she would have lots of ultrasounds because *women carrying twins frequently have sonograms every few weeks after the first trimester.* Finally, Susan brought Karen to a small waiting room filled with books and magazines about having multiples and encouraged her to borrow any of the reading material and to read as much as she could about having twins.

Marie, the nutritionist, then went over Karen's nutritional goals. *Good nutrition is very important for all pregnancies and especially important when carrying multiples,* Marie told her to keep track of what she ate over the next few days. This would help Marie determine if Karen needed to make dietary changes. Marie explained that the *expected weight gain for mothers carrying twins or higher-order multiples is at least five to 10 pounds more* than for a mother carrying a single baby. *Food high in nutritional value,* such as vegetables and fruits, enriched grains, protein, and milk products should total about *2700 calories per day.* She said Karen would need to take *extra vitamins, iron, and folic acid,* as prescribed by Dr. Nelson. Marie then measured Karen's weight and height and recorded them on a chart and in Karen's notebook.

Karen complained that she was suffering from morning sickness, and Marie told her that that *morning sickness can last longer for mothers carrying multiples,* and that for some the sickness continues through the entire pregnancy. But she offered Karen a drink supplement that might ease the nausea and encouraged her to eat frequent snacks, especially before she went to bed—to provide her body with carbohydrates and protein to digest while she slept. She said that keeping high protein carbohydrates with her at all times—granola bars, cheese crackers, or containers of low fat cottage cheese or yogurt in the refrigerator at her office—would also help reduce Karen's nausea. Karen left the office with another appointment scheduled in two weeks and a shopping bag full of educational material. She was tired but felt well cared for.

Why Pregnancy with Multiples Is High Risk

If you're carrying more than one baby during your pregnancy, you are more likely to develop complications. Being pregnant with multiples, for example, can give rise to health complications such as anemia, gestational diabetes, pregnancy induced hypertension (PIH), and intrauterine growth restriction (IUGR). We'll describe these complications in the next chapter. For now, we'll focus on the fact that having a complication of pregnancy often provokes preterm labor and, if undetected or uncontrolled, can lead to the premature birth of your babies.

If you're carrying twins, you have nearly a 50 percent—or one in two—chance of delivering prematurely.[6] Many health care professionals also believe that multiples deliver early because the uterus starts contracting when the babies and other pregnancy material reach a certain weight and size or begin to overstretch the uterus.

Carrying more than one baby in a pregnancy increases the likelihood that your babies will be of low birth weight. Your body may have difficulty accommodating two or more approximately $6^1/2$-pound babies at once and therefore delivers before full term. Low birth weight may also occur because your babies' growth slows.

Usually, the growth of twins is about the same as singletons until about 28 to 30 weeks, when their weight gain slows down and begins to lag behind singleton pregnancies of the same gestation. Sometimes this slower growth may occur before 28 weeks gestation. *One-half of all twin births are of low birth weight*—less than 2500 grams, or 5.5 pounds, ounces—and *almost all triplets or higher number multiples are low birth weight.*[7] These incidences of low birth weight may be because of early delivery, because the babies' growth slowed during the later part of the pregnancy, or a combination of both factors.

There are *significant physical and emotional demands* with a pregnancy carrying multiples, as you will see in Karen and Scott's continuing story that follows.

KAREN AND SCOTT'S STORY (CONTINUED)

Middle Pregnancy with Multiples

At 16 weeks of pregnancy, Karen's regular prenatal tests for blood sugar showed elevated levels. She had a longer, more involved *glucose test for diabetes*, which fortunately was negative.

Karen told Dr. Nelson she was having *leg cramps*. The doctor gave her a supply of *calcium supplements* to help with the leg cramps and checked her for any signs of PIH. Karen also complained about being *constipated* and having severe *heartburn*, neither of which she had experienced before. Marie, the nutritionist, told her to stay away from spicy foods, caffeinated products, and fried foods, and to eat at least one serving a day of food high in bran, such as bran cereal.

As Karen was getting up to dress at the end of the appointment, Dr. Nelson asked if she had any other complaints, and Karen burst into tears. She hadn't been sleeping well, she blurted, because she was so hot and she had to get up to go to the bathroom at least once a night. It seemed like none of her new maternity clothes fit, and she felt like a big baby and a huge blob!

Dr. Nelson offered her a tissue and described the *emotional stress* of pregnancy, adding that having twins can be even more stressful. She suggested that Karen try to take naps on weekends and after work. Dr. Nelson explained that the hormones in pregnancy can slightly elevate the mother's body temperature. She said this is particularly true for mothers carrying more than one baby, and thought that wearing lighter nightclothes and drinking cool drinks might ease Karen's uncomfortable warmth. Dr. Nelson asked Susan the nurse to help Karen access a listing of *support groups for mothers of multiples.* Finally, Dr. Nelson gave Karen a list of the symptoms of depression with instructions to call her if she experienced any of them.

Coping with a High-Risk Pregnancy

If you have a pregnancy with multiples, not only will you have to adapt to the notion of providing care and financial support for more than one baby, but getting the babies to arrive healthy may require extra work. You will inevitably have more periods of stress. In addition, if you're placed on bed rest to aid in continuing your pregnancy (see Chapter 9), you must somehow cope with one or more of the following:

- Sudden isolation
- Inactivity
- Fear for the health of your babies
- Managing a household from your bed
- Negotiating an unexpected transfer of responsibilities at your job

All of this has to be managed when you do not feel sick, making it hard to believe the bed rest prescription is even necessary. It will seem that you're being asked to stop doing all the things you are used to doing and just lie down and await the birth of your babies. Some women carrying twins start feeling very tired in their second trimester and welcome the added rest but many find it to be a very trying period in their lives.

KAREN AND SCOTT'S STORY (Continued)

Late Pregnancy

In her sixth month of pregnancy, Karen asked Scott to come with her to her next prenatal appointment. Karen told her nurse Susan, that she was having more backache than usual. Susan attached her to the NST machine that she explained would tell them if she was having uterine contractions, and monitors the babies' heart rates at the same time. Scott and Karen watched the pen working its way across the paper. The line was mostly level but there was the occasional jagged mountain peak as well. The babies' heart rates sounded clear and strong.

Susan returned every 10–15 minutes and looked at the folds of paper collecting on the floor. She counted four contractions. She explained that *women carrying twins often have trouble distinguishing contractions* from the movements of the two babies *and have more contractions than mothers carrying one baby*. Susan reported the four contractions to Dr. Nelson, who reviewed the strip and noticed that the contractions were irregular in pattern.

Dr. Nelson then examined Karen's cervix and found that it was a little soft but less than one centimeter dilated. She explained to Karen and Scott that the four contractions would be *a baseline for uterine contractions*. This meant that Karen could have *up to four contractions per hour* before the doctor would try to slow the contractions.

As an added precaution, Dr. Nelson suggested it was time for Karen to go on *modified bed rest*. Karen would have to take a leave from her full-time job. Susan explained how to comply with the order for modified bed rest and reviewed with them a list of the signs and symptoms of preterm labor. She urged Karen not to hesitate to call the office to report any new sensations, however minor they seemed. Karen made an appointment to return to the office in one week.

Karen stayed on modified bed rest for the remainder of her pregnancy. She and Scott struggled to adjust their lives to Karen being on bed rest, but they knew that having the babies early was not worth the risk. Karen talked regularly with Susan, who had some good suggestions about how to deal with bed rest. They also enlisted family, friends, and community resources to help them with the household management.

Karen delivered two healthy boys at 37 weeks. The combination of bed rest, Dr. Nelson's close medical care, information and support from Susan, and Scott and Karen's determination, gave Karen's babies the time they needed to grow inside the womb.

Learning all you can from your doctor about your pregnancy with multiples will go a long way toward making you feel more in control of your situation. Here are a few things you can do:

- Ask your doctor for printed information on your condition.
- Study Chapter 5 for the signs and symptoms of preterm labor to be sure you know what to look for and what symptoms to report to your doctor.
- Get support from women who have already given birth to multiples. They will be able to tell you about their experiences with pregnancy and give you an idea of what it will be like once the babies are born. If you have Internet access, there are a number of support sites and chat rooms for women pregnant with multiples.

Avoiding or Delaying Bed Rest

Realistically, when you are pregnant with multiples you will probably have some activity restrictions. To delay them and avoid bed rest, there are several things you can try:

- Get as much rest as possible, including cutting your work hours and taking naps on the weekend and after work.
- Try to avoid stressful situations. Don't overdo it with walking, housework, stair climbing, or heavy lifting.
- Be vigilant about getting enough fluids every day.
- Know the signs and symptoms of preterm labor and PIH.

- Contact your doctor if you experience anything you think may be a problem.

These measures may preserve your energy and stamina and let you remain up and active a little longer, or even for the whole pregnancy. But remember: Bed rest is not a punishment, it is a treatment to help rest your body. *The goal each day is to get one more day in the womb for your babies and one less day in the NICU.* Make a promise to yourself that if your OB Provider wants you on bed rest you won't fight it and you'll do your best to get though this temporary detour in your pregnancy journey.

Home Uterine Activity Monitors

To help your doctor monitor your pregnancy, you may be equipped with a home contraction monitor to detect the number of contractions you're having. Always follow the specific instructions given by your doctor.

Usually you'll be asked to drink a large glass of water to aid in emptying your bladder. Then, you will need to lie down with the monitor attached to your abdomen with belts. You'll probably be asked to do this twice a day. The contraction monitor records the number of contractions you have in a half-hour period and sends this information through the telephone to your doctor's office or to a special contact center that provides your doctor with this information. The nurse who reviews this uterine activity will get to know you and be familiar with your baseline for contractions. She'll call if she feels you're having too many contractions and will give you further instructions depending on the doctor's orders.

Frequent Phone Calls from the Nurse

Many OB providers feel periodic contact with an OB nurse can be helpful. Because of this, many OB providers have a designated OB nurse call you on a regular basis to ask you about possible signs and symptoms of preterm labor or PIH, to see how you're doing with bed rest and medications, and to offer advice and support.

This service proactively reminds you to pay attention to the subtle signs of preterm labor and other complications. Again, most women subconsciously don't want to admit that anything could be wrong because they don't want to be thought of as a worrier or they are afraid that new symptoms may mean worse problems for their pregnancy. These nurses encourage you to communicate how you are feeling physically and emotionally and can offer tips on alleviating the discomforts and isolation. (See Chapter 9 for other tips on how to get through activity reductions and bed rest.)

Visiting Nurses

Occasionally, you may also have the services of a visiting nurse, particularly if you're on strict bed rest. Your doctor doesn't want to risk having you get up out of bed too often which may cause contractions but he or she does want precise prenatal information. This information may include your vital signs, how you're doing on the medication, how many contractions you're having, and how the babies are doing. This information is gleaned from a portable doppler, NST machine or from a portable ultrasound machine.

If your condition is not stable at home, you may be transferred to the hospital to complete your pregnancy.

Being Born Early

About half of sets of twins are born at 36 weeks or earlier, and half of sets of triplets or higher-order multiples arrive before 32 weeks gestation.[7] The majority of these early deliveries are caused by:

- Acute preterm labor
- Maternal hypertension such as PIH, which is a danger to both mother and babies
- Fetal growth restriction—the babies are lagging in growth
- Placental abruption, which means the placenta has separated from the uterine wall and is bleeding

Delivering Multiples

Twins can be delivered vaginally when both babies are head down, but this is rare. Vaginal delivery of both twins will depend upon the position of the babies, their condition, and the expertise of the doctor delivering.

Occasionally, the first twin will be delivered vaginally and then the second twin will need a cesarean. This may happen because the second baby cannot be moved to a head down position, has fetal distress, a prolapsed cord, or because of arrested labor.

Some doctors attempt to turn the second baby (version) and deliver it vaginally. The ideal length of time between delivering the first and second baby should be less than 30 minutes but will also depend on the condition of the second baby. See Chapter 7 for descriptions of both vaginal and cesarean deliveries.

Some circumstances require a cesarean for both babies. Triplets and higher-order multiples are delivered by cesarean. Other circumstances that require a cesarean include:

- Malpresentation of the first baby (breech)
- Placenta previa
- A previous cesarean

Most hospitals today are equipped to handle complicated deliveries and to sustain babies that are fragile. Neonatal specialists have the means and knowledge to resolve most complications and help your babies go home as soon as possible.

Your goal is to stay focused on what is best for you and your babies and to get as much support as you need.

Having a pregnancy with twins or higher-order multiples is difficult and stressful. *You belong to a special group of parents.* You want to do everything to protect your babies. Be assured that there are people willing to help you keep your unborn babies healthy, and who will continue to support you as you begin your new lives together. You and your partner are your babies' heroes!

11

Unexpected Detours on Your Pregnancy Journey

Problems That Can Develop

 Marcia's Journal

> *Dear Journal,*
>   *Having diabetes is no big deal anymore. I was really scared with my first pregnancy, but the doctors and nurses assured me everything should be fine if I followed their directions. They were right! Chris is three and a half, and Josh is due in another week. Having diabetes is a pain but something I have to live with. Now I know that if I take my illness in stride and keep my mind on the outcome, my pregnancies are fine.*

During your pregnancy, your OB provider has been on the lookout for signs and symptoms that your body may be having difficulties. This vigilance has ensured that any problems that arise are taken care of as soon as they're detected. Early treatment helps prevent problems from worsening and leading to other complications.

You may have developed a complication that requires special care by your OB provider. Whatever the circumstance or situation, if you've developed a pregnancy complication, you can help protect your pregnancy by learning about it. Learning about and understanding your condition and what's happening to you and your baby will empower you to work with your OB provider to maintain a safe pregnancy and minimize any adverse effects on your baby's health and your own. Follow your OB provider's instructions for your care, because this will help you in your effort to protect your pregnancy.

Ideally, your baby will remain in the womb until full term, but some complications of pregnancy will mean that your baby will be better off being born early, which means that your pregnancy will end and your baby will be delivered. The outcome of your complicated pregnancy is usually improved when you report any changes in your physical well-being, see your health care provider regularly, and follow his or her recommendations. Your health care providers are well versed in how to treat problems and to determine what's best for you and your baby.

The Complications of Pregnancy

Developing a complication during your pregnancy may make it high risk. You may experience preterm labor, and your baby may have to be delivered early. Your care may be put under the charge of a perinatologist, a highly trained medical specialist for high-risk pregnancies whose goal is to eliminate—or at least minimize—any secondary problems caused by the complication, and to maintain your pregnancy and the health of your baby.

When complications are detected early and controlled through close observation and proper medical management, premature birth may be avoided, and you'll most likely have a healthy outcome for yourself and your baby.

If you are diagnosed with one of the complications of pregnancy we'll discuss below, you will certainly receive detailed explanations from your doctor, and you may also be given patient education brochures and other printed literature to help you understand what has happened to your pregnancy. Of course, check with your doctor about where you can also seek out reliable information on the Internet to supplement your knowledge.

The following thumbnail descriptions will provide an outline of your condition. They may also be helpful to your concerned friends and family—those who wish to understand what's happened to your pregnancy.

Incompetent Cervix

If you have an "incompetent cervix," your cervix is not able to remain closed during the pregnancy. Sometimes it lacks the normal firmness or it can also be very short. From about 13 weeks of pregnancy, the combined weight of the baby, the fluids, and the placenta may exert enough pressure on the cervix to cause it to thin and open, resulting in a miscarriage.

Miscarriage from an incompetent cervix may occur as early as the fourteenth week of pregnancy if undetected or untreated. When incompetent cervix affects a pregnancy after the twentieth week of gestation, it can lead to preterm labor and birth.

Diagnosing Cervical Incompetence

In the past, your incompetent cervix might not have been diagnosed until you'd had several miscarriages. Nowadays, physicians can check for this problem after one miscarriage. Vaginal ultrasound detects early changes in the cervix. An incompetent cervix can be treated with a minor surgical procedure that is somewhat like putting a sewing stitch through the cervix. This procedure, called *cerclage*, will be described in more detail in the following paragraphs.

DES and Incompetent Cervix

You may have an incompetent cervix because your mother took *diethylstilbestrol (DES)* during her pregnancy with you. From 1938 to 1971, many women took the medication DES to prevent miscarriages during their pregnancies. It was later discovered that their daughters often had defects in their reproductive organs.

Having an abnormally shaped uterus or cervix can cause you to miscarry due to incompetent cervix. If you are the daughter of a woman who used DES, you may have:

- *Abnormalities of the uterus.* A *bicornuate* uterus is heart-shaped, and a *didelphic* uterus is one that has two compartments, separated by a wall, in the uterus. Often with a didelphic uterus there are two cervices. Both abnormalities can prevent a fetus from growing but are correctable. An *underdeveloped cervix* opens prematurely and requires surgical intervention to maintain pregnancy.

- *Abnormal pap smears*. The cells on the surface of the cervix are not normal and indicate the possibility that cervical cancer may develop.

Happily, over time there will be fewer and fewer women with malformed reproductive organs due to DES because the use of this medication was stopped in 1971. The youngest women affected by this medication are in their mid-30s in the first decade of the 2000s.

FACTS

The National Cancer Institute wants to alert women who took DES between 1938 and 1971 about additional dangers of DES exposure. You should be aware that:

- You should contact your mother and grandmother to see if there is a chance they took DES while pregnant. DES-exposed women are at an increased risk for breast cancer.
- Daughters of women who took DES should know that they're at increased risk for infertility and a rare form of vaginal cancer called "clear cell cancer." The National Cancer Institute says all DES daughters need special care during pregnancy.
- The institute also advises DES sons to be on the lookout for benign cysts on the back of the testicles, for underdeveloped testicles, and for an increased risk of infertility.[1]

Other Causes

Having a mother who took DES is not the only reason you may have cervical incompetence; there are other conditions that may cause this complication of pregnancy.

Previous surgery on the cervix may cause cervical incompetence. *Conization* surgically removes a wedge of the internal part of the cervix to treat cervical cancer. Or *loop electrosurgical excision procedure* (LEEP) might be used, in which a wire loop sends an electrical current to the surface of the cervix to remove precancerous cells. Unfortunately, these necessary procedures are currently being researched to determine if there is a link to possible causes of incompetent cervix.

It is also speculated that frequent elective abortions may lead to cervical incompetence. Because the cervix must be dilated manually during an elective abortion, the ability of the cervical muscle to maintain its ability to remain closed during pregnancy can decrease. However, medical literature does not state how many elective abortions can cause cervical incompetence.

Sometimes the cause of an incompetent cervix cannot be determined, but treatment for this condition, whether or not the cause is known, is very effective for most women. Most can expect to have an otherwise healthy pregnancy once measures are in place to keep your cervix closed until time for delivery.

Cerclage

Incompetent cervix is often treated with the above-mentioned surgical procedure called a cerclage (pronounced "ser-klahsh"). In this operation, your doctor puts several surgical stitches into the cervix. The stitches act like a "purse string" to reinforce the cervix and keep it from opening too soon.

The procedure is done between the fourteenth and twentieth week of pregnancy and is performed in the operating room at the hospital under anesthesia. Recovery time is usually short; in most cases you are discharged the same day. You may experience some mild cramping and spotting after you get home. You should call your doctor if the cramping or bleeding does not stop after a few days. Occasionally, your doctor may prescribe medications to prevent infection and to stop the cramping.

There are two types of cerclage. The most frequently performed is the *McDonald cerclage*. With this procedure, the temporary cerclage stitches are removed at full term to allow for the vaginal birth of your baby. If you've had a very difficult time with miscarriages because of the incompetent cervix, your doctor may perform a *Shirodkar* cerclage. With this procedure, the cerclage stitches are more or less permanent and your baby is delivered by cesarean section.

Hourglass Membranes

Your cervix may be so weak that the amniotic sac or membrane drops into your cervical canal. These are called "hourglass membranes" because the amniotic sac begins to look like an hourglass, with wide areas in the uterus and in the cervical canal. The narrow cervix in the middle completes the hourglass shape. This condition is treated in the hospital. Your hospital bed will be put into the Trendelenberg position, meaning your head will be lower than your feet. Over a period of a day or two, gravity allows the membranes to slide back up into the uterus before cerclage stitches are placed in the cervix.

Uterine Fibroids

Fibroids are benign growths of muscle tissue. They're also called *myomas* or *leiomyomas*. Uterine fibroids occur in 20 to 25 percent of all women, most commonly in women 30 to 40 years of age. They appear in all groups of women, but seem to have a higher incidence among African Americans.[2]

You may be unaware you have fibroids until you're pregnant. They are diagnosed during a pelvic exam or with ultrasound. Even in pregnancy, your fibroids may not cause any problems. Complications occur when they grow large enough to compete with the fetus for space in the uterus. Some women experience fibroid pain caused by the growth of the fibroid impinging on the uterine cavity. This pain is sometimes treated with anti-inflammatory agents.

The hormone estrogen increases rapidly in the early months of pregnancy and can stimulate some fibroids to grow very large. In early pregnancy, fibroids can cause a miscarriage. In later pregnancy, crowding from the fibroids can cause the uterus to begin contracting and lead to preterm labor and premature birth. If the fibroids are growing across the cervical opening, a cesarean delivery may be necessary.

Preterm Premature Rupture of Membranes

PPROM is a complication that can cause miscarriage before 20 weeks of pregnancy or premature delivery after 20 weeks. It is estimated that *one-third of preterm labor cases are caused by preterm premature rupture of the membranes*.[3] This significant prenatal complication may also occur without preterm labor.

When premature rupture occurs, you must be sent to the hospital immediately, regardless of whether you are in labor. Your doctor will

NANETTE'S STORY

Nanette was at her 24-week checkup when her doctor told her hat she had a fibroid that was becoming quite large—about the size of an orange—and that it could possibly cause problems in her pregnancy. The doctor explained that the fibroid was down close to the opening of her cervix and might prevent it from opening enough to have a vaginal delivery. The fibroid might also provoke preterm labor contractions. She felt Nanette should prepare herself for the possibility that she would need a cesarean delivery.

Nanette asked what could be done about the fibroid. The doctor explained that she couldn't remove the fibroid but that she would check it at each prenatal visit using ultrasound. She wanted Nanette to be sure to report any unusual symptoms or changes in her pregnancy.

Nanette went home and told her husband about this complication of her pregnancy. She decided to read up on fibroids to have a better idea of what to watch for. She memorized the signs and symptoms of preterm labor and also learned about having a cesarean. About two weeks later, Nanette noticed cramping and an uncomfortable pulling sensation where her doctor told her the fibroid was located. On examination, her doctor told her everything was fine and the pain was caused by the growth of the fibroid. She told her to try ibuprofen every 4 to 6 hours and to get more rest. The pain recurred on and off for about three more weeks and then stopped. At 36 weeks she went into labor and, indeed, needed to be delivered by cesarean section. But Nanette felt prepared, and so was calm during the procedure. She delivered Kyla, a healthy baby girl.

try to establish why the PPROM occurred and determine if delivery is imminent. When PPROM occurs many weeks before your baby is due, there is a risk of infection as well as the risk of early delivery.

What Causes PPROM?

A diagnosis of PPROM means the membranes surrounding the fetus have weakened and lost their elasticity. Just what causes this weakening is uncertain, but there's some speculation that a bacterial infection is the culprit. In the past, preterm premature rupture of the membranes meant immediate delivery because the risk of acquiring an infection was thought to be high. Because some women did not deliver immediately after PPROM and did not develop an infection, today the more common approach is to wait and see how you and your baby do.

If your baby is near 26 weeks gestation or more, when there is a good chance of surviving, the goal is to delay the delivery long enough to give you a course of corticosteroids to stimulate your baby's lungs to mature more quickly. Delivery may be successfully postponed anywhere from a few hours to a few weeks, but the remainder of the pregnancy must be closely supervised in a hospital setting and with bed rest. Surprisingly, some women have gotten two to three months further into their pregnancies before delivering, but this is not the norm.

Treatment

Treatment of PPROM varies according to the amount of fluid remaining in the amniotic sac, the gestational age of the baby, and whether you're at risk for infection.

A sample of your vaginal fluid is collected and cultured to see if infection is present. Results take from 24 to 48 hours. You may be started on antibiotics immediately while waiting for the results of the tests since most women in the early stages of infection do not exhibit any symptoms. Your doctor will probably measure the amount of fluid remaining in the womb using ultrasound. If there is sufficient fluid, the pregnancy can be maintained. A small tear, called a "high leak" because it occurs in the upper half of the uterus, usually lets out only a small amount of amniotic fluid. However, even a small amniotic fluid leak can progress into continuous leaking and initiate labor.

Sometimes a small tear in the sac heals on its own. If this happens, your pregnancy will probably continue to a full-term delivery. Your doctor will monitor your condition because you are still at risk for infection. Most often, you will be allowed to go home with a prescription for bed rest. If you have signs of a mild infection, your doctor will probably keep you in the hospital and try to treat the infection. However, if infection occurs, your doctor may feel it is safer for your baby to be delivered promptly.

Infections

When a serious infection is confirmed, most doctors agree that your baby should be delivered within 12 hours despite its prematurity. A further complication for PPROM is that if your bag of water or amniotic sac ruptures without contractions and thus without changes to the cervix, your doctor may try inducing labor, but delivery will probably have to be by cesarean.

Infection of the amniotic fluid may lead to PPROM or may cause its own complications in pregnancy. For reasons not yet understood, bacteria that is normally found in the fluid of the vagina begins to multiply and sometimes crosses into the uterus. These bacteria can also spread to the amniotic sac and the baby. The bacteria must be treated with antibiotics before they proliferate in the uterine cavity.

The most commonly found types of invading bacteria are: Group Beta streptococcus (GBS), bacterial vaginosis (BV), which we'll discuss below; Ureaplasma urealyticum, Mycoplasma hominis, Gardnerella vaginalis, peptostreptococcus, bacteriodes species, trichomonas, and Chlamydia trachomatis.

BETH'S STORY

Beth, age 34 and living in Boulder, Colorado, miscarried her first pregnancy at nine weeks. Her second pregnancy continued normally to the seventh month, when she woke up one night and discovered the sheets soaked with clear fluid. In the bathroom, Beth noticed tiny spots of blood on her toilet tissue. At the hospital, her doctor diagnosed PPROM.

Beth remained in the hospital under observation for four days. Every day the nurses checked her vital signs and drew blood to check for infection. They also monitored her baby's heart rate and Beth's contractions with the fetal monitor. On the fifth day, she began to feel ill and was told her temperature was elevated. The doctor determined that she had an infection and decided to induce labor. She delivered a 31-week-old baby girl who weighed only three pounds. Her baby required oxygen and antibiotics for infection, and remained in the hospital for five weeks. Her daughter, Angelina, recovered and became a healthy, normal baby.

Group B Beta Hemolytic Streptococcus

One common microbe that may complicate a diagnosis of PPROM is Group B Strep bacteria (GBS). GBS is a normal organism in your body; however, sometimes during pregnancy it can proliferate and lead to acute infections in the vagina, cervix, or urinary tract. Most women don't have the common symptoms of this bacterial infection, which include a fever, or feeling achy, and fatigued.

The March of Dimes reports (from the CDC) that 10 to 30 percent of pregnant women carry the GBS bacterium, but most experience no illness.[4] If your OB provider feels you may have GBS, you will probably not receive antibiotics immediately after the diagnosis. Most health care providers agree that women with GBS should not be treated with antibiotics during the earlier part of their pregnancy as long as they have no symptoms of preterm labor and there is no evidence of PPROM.

Screening for GBS. Currently all women are cultured for GBS between the thirty-fifth and thirty-seventh week of pregnancy. Previously, women were cultured early in their pregnancy. If the results were positive, they were treated. Unfortunately, the rate of reinfection was very high. Because the medical community is concerned that overuse of antibiotics can make the immune system unresponsive to treatment later, when it can be critical, nowadays testing and treatment is delayed to closer to delivery time.

Treatment of GBS. If you are full-term, you will be given the antibiotics during early labor, before you deliver your baby. If you are hospitalized because a premature birth seems likely, you will be tested and treated for GBS infection immediately upon your arrival if you are in preterm labor, have PPROM, or have had a previous child infected with GBS. Having GBS is relatively harmless for you, but you'll need to be treated because GBS can cause serious health problems for your baby after it's born.

The treatment for GBS is intravenous (IV) antibiotics, because oral medication is not thought to be as effective. It also appears that the antibiotics are far more effective if they are in your system 4–5 hours before delivery. If you are full term and tested positive at your GBS screening, most OB Providers may instruct you to come to the hospital or birthing center in early labor to start you on IV antibiotics. This gives the medication time to circulate in you and your baby's systems.

How GBS Can Hurt the Baby. GBS in babies can occur when they come in contact with vaginal fluid that contains the bacteria during a vaginal birth. If the bacteria gets into the baby's respiratory or digestive system, the baby may contract GBS. It does not appear that skin contact alone is harmful.

Babies with GBS can develop pneumonia, a blood infection called *sepsis*, or *meningitis*, an infection of the membranes around the brain. These are all potentially dangerous conditions requiring intensive care and can result in death.

Babies with GBS are classified as either early or late onset. *Early onset* means they show signs of infection within seven days of birth, and most of these babies exhibit symptoms within six hours of birth. *Late onset* occurs between seven days and three months after birth.

GBS infection can be especially difficult for a preterm infant. Fortunately, the incidence of this for all babies, full term and preterm, has dropped 70 percent since health care providers began providing antibiotic treatment during labor and delivery. Today, thanks to surveillance and prompt action by obstetrics providers, GBS now infects only about one in 2000 babies each year. This number is certain to decrease even further over time.[5]

Bacterial Vaginosis

Bacterial vaginosis (pronounced "vaj-i-noh-sis"), or BV, is another type of bacteria commonly found in small, harmless amounts in the vagina. When the protective and beneficial bacteria lactobacillus diminishes, the vagina becomes alkaline, and the alkaline vagina allows for an increased growth in harmful levels of BV bacteria. A BV infection can lead to preterm labor.

The number of pregnant women who have *dangerous* levels of BV is thought to be as high as 16 percent.[6] You may be more familiar with other names for BV, like Gardnerella vaginitis, nonspecific vaginitis, or Haemophilus vaginitis.

BV is treated with antibiotics. The most effective medication is Metronidazole, also called Flagyl. It is usually not given until the second trimester.

FACTS ABOUT BACTERIAL VAGINOSIS

- May cause a strong fishy odor from the vagina, especially after intercourse
- May cause a thin, gray or pale whitish discharge
- Usually does not cause itching, burning, or pain of any kind

Chorioamnionitis

One rarer kind of infection, *chorioamnionitis*, affects the chorion—the layer between the amniotic sac and the uterus. Often there are no symptoms of this infection in its early stages.

If your health care provider suspects that you might have chorioamnionitis, he or she will be on the lookout for:

- Uterine tenderness, meaning the uterus is painful when touched.
- Uterus feels hard and possibly swollen when touched although contractions aren't occurring
- Mild fever (100.1° F.)
- General aches and pains, malaise
- Rapid heartbeat in the unborn baby or in you

TIP

You can help monitor your condition by reporting any unusual or new symptoms during your pregnancy. Early testing will enable your OB provider to begin early treatment. Treating infections with antibiotics is a very effective way of preventing preterm labor and premature birth.

Placenta Previa

Your placenta supplies the baby with nutrients through the umbilical cord. In most cases, the placenta attaches to the upper wall of the uterus. If you're diagnosed with *placenta previa*, your placenta is developing low in the uterus, where it can be easily damaged. In some cases the placenta starts off low in the uterus but as the lower segment of the uterus expands, the placenta is in a higher position and is no longer a potential source of trouble for your pregnancy.

There are often no symptoms of placenta previa. It may be discovered by chance during an ultrasound exam, or occasionally there is painless bleeding from the vagina, usually late in the pregnancy. *Bleeding at any time in your pregnancy should be reported immediately to your OB provider.*

Most women with placenta previa have only a little vaginal spotting or bleeding. However, if you have heavy bleeding because of this condition, you may hemorrhage; that is, lose a dangerous amount of blood. Hemorrhaging also deprives your baby of oxygen. You may need blood transfusions, and your baby may need to be delivered quickly.

Placenta previa occurs in about one out of 200 pregnancies and is rare in first pregnancies.[7] If you have had cesareans or other abdominal surgery or are carrying multiples, you're more likely to experience placenta previa.

There are three types of placenta previa (see Figure 11-1):

1. A *complete previa* means the placenta is completely over the cervix. A complete previa will require cesarean delivery because the baby cannot pass the placenta and the pushing and pressure of the baby's head will cause significant bleeding.

2. A *partial or marginal previa* means the placenta is partially covering the cervix. This kind of previa needs to be evaluated by the doctor at the time of delivery but many times the baby is delivered by cesarean.

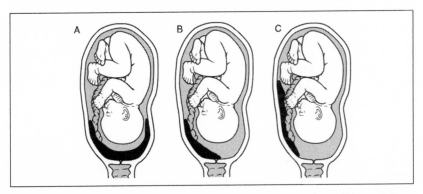

FIGURE 11-1 Three types of placenta previa: (A) complete, (B) partial, and (C) low-lying.

3. A *low-lying placenta* means the placenta is near the opening of the cervix. This condition only becomes a problem when the baby cannot move down into the birth canal without causing trauma to the placenta and thus bleeding.

Treatment for Placenta Previa

Even with very little bleeding or spotting from the previa, your doctor will have to monitor you very closely. This will mean frequent sonograms to check on the position of your placenta. Cervical exams are limited because they can provoke bleeding. You will be restricted from having intercourse. If the placenta is only covering the cervix partially, you may be able to deliver vaginally.

If you have a complete placenta previa, you're usually put on strict bed rest and you may have to be hospitalized for part of your pregnancy, especially if you start to have bleeding. When your baby is full term, you will probably be delivered by cesarean. The doctor may decide to perform the cesarean before your labor starts to avoid the possible complications of bleeding or to avoid an emergency cesarean.

Pregnancy-Induced Hypertension

Your health depends on many things, but one system it particularly depends on is your circulatory system.

Your heart pumps blood through the blood vessels. When these blood vessels become smaller because the inside layer of muscle is contracting, less blood can get through the system. Then the heart has to work harder to pump blood. When this occurs, the pressure in the blood vessels increases and you can develop high blood pressure. Small fluctuations in blood pressure are normal and occur in everyone throughout each day. When blood pressure remains above normal for extended periods, health care providers become concerned about your cardiovascular system.

There are two types of high blood pressure for pregnant women. Some women have high blood pressure before they became pregnant, which is called *chronic hypertension*. Others develop *pregnancy-induced hypertension*, or PIH, which, as the name implies, is high blood pressure developed during pregnancy.

Cause of PIH

The cause of PIH is not yet known, but some researchers speculate it may occur because your body is seeing the components of pregnancy, such as the baby's different blood type or different genetic makeup, as unfamiliar and is defending itself. The problems with PIH usually don't occur until the thirteenth week of pregnancy, when your body will start reacting to these components. However, the actual PIH *symptoms* don't manifest themselves until after the twentieth week of pregnancy. The symptoms can be mild to severe.

Another theory of the cause of PIH has to do with pregnancy hormones. Normally in pregnancy, hormones relax the muscles and blood vessels. This does not occur in women with PIH. For some reason their bodies do not respond to the hormonal influence. The blood vessels are persistently contracted causing higher pressure within the vessels and the heart must work harder causing an elevation in blood pressure.

If you develop high blood pressure in your pregnancy, your doctor will be concerned about both you and your baby. Your baby's development and health depends on your circulatory system, which supplies needed nutrients and oxygen. Having high blood pressure can affect your health as well.

Symptoms

PIH symptoms may be mild to severe. They include:

- Water retention, bloating, and swelling in hands and face
- Double vision, blurred vision, or frequent spots in your vision, like a camera flash in your eyes
- Mild elevation of blood pressure, 130/90 to 140/90
- Headaches that are not resolved with acetaminophen
- Weight gain of more than one pound a day
- Protein in your urine (when checked at your prenatal appointment)
- Pressure or pain in the upper right side of your abdomen

Many women who have never had high blood pressure and have no risk factors for high blood pressure develop PIH during pregnancy, so doctors and midwives check for signs of it at every prenatal appointment.

Who Is at Risk?

Women who appear to be at heightened risk for this condition are those:

- Who are pregnant for the first time
- Who are carrying multiples
- Over 40 years old
- With problems such as heart disease, diabetes, and kidney disease
- With autoimmune diseases like lupus
- With a history of high blood pressure
- With a family history of high blood pressure or PIH
- Who are African American

TRY THIS

If you're diagnosed with PIH:

- See your doctor regularly. Report any change in PIH symptoms.
- Report any other conditions you may have, such as kidney disease or diabetes.
- Report all medications you're taking.
- Find ways to check your blood pressure between doctor visits, at an employee health center, for instance, or through a neighbor with a self-blood-pressure kit or a machine at the local grocery store. Record your blood pressures and take these numbers to your doctor visits.
- Get a scale to weigh yourself at home regularly, preferably at the same time every day. Keep a log of your weekly weight.
- Drink water throughout the day and rest with your legs elevated frequently, especially when you first get home from work or in the evening.

Preeclampsia

Pregnancy-induced hypertension can develop into preeclampsia. Preeclampsia warns doctors that your body is not handling the pregnancy well and is a precondition of the toxic state called eclampsia, or *toxemia*. These days, full-blown eclampsia is rare because at every prenatal appointment OB providers check for its precursors—PIH and preeclampsia—and they take prompt action to prevent your condition from worsening.

Preeclampsia can make your kidney, liver, or other organs malfunction normally. It can also weaken the muscles of your heart. When blood pressure remains high for extended periods, your kidneys cannot process wastes as efficiently and begin to spill protein into the urine. Detecting protein in the urine is another way to diagnose PIH and preeclampsia.

Preeclampsia is also potentially harmful to your baby because, as we mentioned above, high blood pressure means less oxygen is available for the baby's development. Your baby may remain much smaller than he or she should be for its gestational age. This condition is called *intrauterine growth restricted*, or IUGR. This means that your baby's growth is being slowed down by the lack of oxygen. If your baby's growth seems to be slowing, he or she will be monitored frequently using ultrasound and fetal heart monitoring. We'll discuss IUGR further below.

Symptoms of Preeclampsia

- Extreme swelling in hands, knees, and face
- Rapid weight gain
- Increased protein in the urine (shown in testing)
- Elevated blood pressure (over 140/90)
- Problems with vision: blurring, light dots, aversion to bright light
- Severe or constant headaches unrelieved by acetaminophen
- Pressure in the lower chest between the ribs or upper right of abdomen
- Nausea and vomiting

Treatment for Preeclampsia
To help yourself and your baby when you have preeclampsia:

- Reduce salt intake.
- Drink 8–10 glasses of water a day.
- Get a blood pressure monitoring kit and chart results daily to take to your OB visits.
- Maintain a diet high in protein. Avoid fried, high-calorie, and nonnutritious foods.

- Get plenty of rest, or maintain bed rest if recommended by your doctor.
- Lie on your side as much as possible. Try to favor the left side to increase the blood supply to the uterus and thus to the baby.
- When sitting, elevate your feet, but avoid forming a right angle that may impede blood return from the legs to the heart. Avoid tight stockings or clothing that restricts circulation to your legs.
- Avoid alcohol and caffeine.
- Avoid stressful situations.
- Keep track of your baby's movement every day.
- Notify your OB provider immediately if your symptoms of pre-eclampsia worsen or new ones develop.

The treatment for preeclampsia usually involves close monitoring of your blood pressure and looking for protein in your urine. You may be equipped with devices that allow you to measure these symptoms at home. Your doctor will recommend bed rest with plenty of fluids because it may help decrease stress and allow your body to recover on its own. He or she will also ask you to come into the office more frequently to monitor your baby's heart rate and movements and to measure the amniotic fluid inside your uterus.

If these treatments do not work and your condition does not improve, you may need to be hospitalized for closer continuous monitoring of your baby and may be treated with intravenous medication.

Intrauterine Growth Restriction

When the placenta does not supply enough nourishment and oxygen to the developing baby, the baby's growth is delayed. This is called intrauterine growth restriction, and it may be caused by high blood pressure, preeclampsia, antepartum hemorrhage, placenta previa, heart disease, severe malnutrition, or diabetes mellitus.

Sometimes, decreased fetal movement or slow growth of the uterus signals IUGR. Since decreased fetal movement can suggest a wide range of problems, it's important to inform the doctor as soon as possible if there is a change in how often your baby moves. The doctor will probably perform an ultrasound to measure the size of the baby. If growth is delayed, bed rest and a change of diet may be recommended to improve the baby's weight and growth. In some cases, your doctor may decide on an early delivery because the environment outside of the uterus (the intensive care nursery) is more controlled than inside of the uterus. This allows the baby to continue developing by ensuring that the baby is getting adequate nourishment.

At birth, a baby who is IUGR, whether full term or not, may have little body fat to keep it warm and may have some of the complications of prematurity, such as respiratory distress syndrome. Once delivered, these babies usually respond quickly and positively to supplemental oxygen and nutrients, fattening up or gaining weight to a normal baby size and acquiring a healthy pink glow.

Anemia

A vital component of blood, *hemoglobin*, carries oxygen throughout the body. You need the nutrients iron and folic acid to produce hemoglobin, and being pregnant alters the normal processes of the digestive system so that these nutrients may pass through without being absorbed. When not enough hemoglobin is present, anemia results.

The symptoms of anemia include:

- Paleness
- Weakness
- Tiredness
- Breathlessness
- Fainting
- Palpitations, or a sensation that your heart is beating very fast

If insufficient absorption of iron is not the problem, diet may be the cause of your anemia. You may not be eating foods that are high in iron and folic acid. See Chapter 3 for a listing of iron-rich foods.

If you are getting enough iron in your diet but still have anemia, the usual course of treatment is to take iron supplements with ascorbic acid (vitamin C) in addition to your prenatal vitamin, to try to boost the iron level of your blood. The vitamin C helps your body digest the iron. However, the iron tablets may still be hard to digest and may cause indigestion or constipation, especially in the first trimester when morning sickness is a factor. This can be alleviated by taking the tablets right after meals, with milk or crushed and put into something like applesauce. In extreme cases, iron may also be given as an injection. With severe anemia, blood transfusions may be needed.

Anemia puts you at risk for having a premature birth and makes you more prone to infection. It may also make you less able to sustain a sudden blood loss during delivery of your baby.

Diabetes and Pregnancy

Some women have diabetes before they get pregnant and some acquire it after becoming pregnant. Your body when pregnant has a higher demand for insulin.

Diabetes is caused when your body's production of *insulin*, a hormone that converts sugar in the blood to energy, malfunctions. Sometimes there is not enough insulin produced or it can't be used effectively to convert the sugar in your blood to energy. As a result, this sugar builds up in your blood. There is no mechanism to off-load or use the sugar, and the symptoms and effects of diabetes occur.

Some women develop diabetes prior to pregnancy. This is called *pregestational diabetes*. This type of diabetes in pregnancy is a challenge to the mother and her physician because of the increased demands that the pregnancy makes on the body. Many of these women are already on supplemental insulin, oral hypoglycemic agents, or controlled diet. These women will probably need to take insulin supplements to control their diabetes while they are pregnant.

The hormones of the placenta can affect your body's production of insulin and lead to what is termed *gestational diabetes*, which first shows up during pregnancy, between the twenty-fourth and twenty-eighth week. Testing for gestational diabetes at weeks 24–28 is a standard in the medical profession because many women do not notice any symptoms.

Those Most Likely to Develop Gestational Diabetes
You're more likely to develop maternal diabetes if you:

- Are obese
- Have high blood pressure
- Have a family history of diabetes
- Are over 30 years old
- Are Hispanic or African American

Symptoms
The symptoms of gestational diabetes include:

- Frequent urination, sometimes as often as every hour
- Excessive thirst
- Fatigue and weakness
- Loss of weight or rapid weight gain
- Tingling in the hands and feet
- Reduced resistance to infections, including urinary tract infections
- Occasional blurred vision
- Glucose or sugar in the urine

Testing for Diabetes
Most pregnant women are checked for abnormal glucose levels at every prenatal visit. However, the standard glucose screening for gestational diabetes is a *1-hour glucose screening* test performed on most women at 24–26 weeks into their pregnancy. You will be asked to drink a sweet soda-like beverage and have your blood drawn one hour later. If your results are elevated, you will be asked to take a three-hour glucose tolerance test (GTT) another day. This is a diagnostic test that confirms gestational diabetes.

In preparation for the three-hour GTT, you'll be asked to consume a carbohydrate-rich diet for the three days before the test and then fast the night before. The next day you'll have blood drawn and then be given another sweet sodalike drink. Your blood will be drawn at regular intervals three more times and tested to find out how much sugar remains in your blood. If your blood is abnormal at the end of the testing period, you have gestational diabetes.

Treating Gestational Diabetes

The glucose tolerance test tells your doctor whether you have diabetes and the severity of the problem. Depending upon these results, you'll either be given a diabetic diet to control your blood sugar and carbohydrate intake or you'll be put on medication immediately along with the diet. Controlling your glucose level is very important to having a healthy pregnancy, delivery, and baby.

Your OB provider may prescribe a self-glucose testing kit that measures your blood glucose levels and will tell you how often to self-test. His or her nurse or staff member will teach you how to use the kit and how to follow a diabetic diet that includes fresh fruit, vegetables, pasta, rice, potatoes, and lean meats. Eating more frequent, smaller meals throughout the day and before bedtime is another important practice.

Exercise is another critical component for controlling diabetes. With regular exercise, your body doesn't need as much insulin to keep blood sugars in check. Your OB provider and staff will help you establish your diet and level of exercise; walking, swimming, and yoga are all good choices to help you control your diabetes in pregnancy.

But if diet and exercise are not effective, if your initial blood sugars are too high, or you're unable to adhere to the regimen, insulin injections or (nowadays) oral hypoglycemic agents may be prescribed. You may need to be hospitalized for a short time to allow your doctor to control your diabetes more precisely and monitor the condition of your baby.

Your OB provider will probably follow your pregnancy more closely and monitor the baby more often as you get closer to full term. You may be referred to a perinatologist, a specialist in high-risk pregnancies, for more specialized care and to a nutritionist for help with your diet. Controlling your diabetes will improve your own health and your baby's health tremendously, and you will be working actively to delay the onset of adult diabetes. It is believed that women with gestational diabetes have a 50 percent chance of developing diabetes again later in life.[8]

The Importance of Well-Controlled Diabetes

Diabetes is usually manageable, but it puts you at greater risk for other complications of pregnancy. These risks include preeclampsia; *polyhydramnios* (an excess fluid in the amniotic sac); and frequent urinary tract infections (UTIs), which are often without symptoms. Untreated UTIs may infect your kidneys, prohibiting them from effectively cleaning toxins from your system.

Having diabetes can also affect your baby's health. Babies born to mothers with uncontrolled pregestational diabetes are more at risk for birth defects. For both pregestational and gestational diabetes, the more common complication is that the excess and unused sugar from your system may go to your baby, making it grow larger than normal. Not only is this large baby more difficult to deliver, but he or she can have hypoglycemia (low blood sugar), excess red blood cells, jaundice, and a physiologically immature respiratory system at birth. Some of these babies require intensive care just after birth, but most babies recover quickly.

You have a good chance of having a vaginal birth even with diabetes. According to the CDC in 2000, 38.4 percent, or more than one-third of women with diabetes, were delivered by cesarean deliveries, but that means two-thirds had vaginal deliveries.[9] You can breast-feed your baby even if you have already been treated for gestational diabetes.

Postpartum Care of Diabetes

Once home with your baby, you should continue your diet and exercise routine, and you may be asked to monitor your glucose levels, since they will be affected by the delivery, nursing, and daily life with your baby. Your gestational diabetes should resolve itself gradually after the baby is born. Make sure your internist or the family practice physician you see for routine care knows you had gestational diabetes and checks your blood sugar periodically, especially if you are planning to have another pregnancy. Preconceptual counseling is critical before becoming pregnant again.

Polyhydramnios

Polyhydramnios is an increase in the amniotic fluid of the amniotic sac. In most cases, this condition develops gradually. Your symptoms— from the excess fluid and enlarged uterus—may include a greater difficulty catching your breath, frequent indigestion, and tightness of the abdomen. In a very few cases, however, the fluid buildup is rapid, you feel nauseous, and you may go into preterm labor.

Polyhydramnios is most often found in women with diabetes, preeclampsia, women who are carrying multiples, or when a baby has a birth defect.

For mild polyhydramnios, doctors usually prescribe extra rest and frequent sonograms to check the baby and measure the fluid. When the onset of polyhydramnios is fast, the doctor will probably prescribe complete bed rest and medications to decrease the fluid. Sometimes the doctor will drain the excess fluid by inserting a needle into the amniotic sac.

Placental Abruption

When the placenta separates from the uterine wall, it's called *placental abruption*. This dangerous condition usually occurs in the last 12 weeks of pregnancy. Symptoms include vaginal bleeding and constant pain in the abdomen. *Report any vaginal bleeding to your OB provider immediately.*

The symptoms of this condition are different from the bleeding caused by a placenta previa. With placental abruption, there is vaginal bleeding as well as severe abdominal pain, a very tender abdomen when touched, and a very firm uterus. When abruption occurs, there are two dangers: decreased oxygen to the baby and maternal hemorrhage. Treatment includes immediate hospitalization, continuous evaluation of the baby, and measures to stop the bleeding. In most cases your baby will have to be delivered immediately. A minor separation may result in a blood clot that stops the bleeding and can be treated and monitored for the remainder of the pregnancy, thus avoiding a premature delivery.

A Loss

Some complications of pregnancy result in the loss of the pregnancy such as a miscarriage or premature birth. Other times your baby can be stillborn. Your OB provider will probably be able to determine what has occurred, explain to you what has happened, and offer you and your partner support for this unexpected and traumatic event.

If you've experienced the loss of a pregnancy, you may find it helpful to talk with others who have had similar experiences. You may also want to seek comfort and understanding from a mental health professional who can help you through this difficult time. After giving yourself enough time to fully grieve for the loss of your baby, you may want to talk to your doctor about trying to get pregnant again.

ANN'S STORY

Ann went on a two-mile walk with her husband Rick. At one point she remembers jumping down from a rock and feeling a sharp twinge in her abdomen. It felt like a pulled muscle. She was about 27 weeks pregnant.

That evening, she began bleeding from her vagina and had Rick take her to the hospital. The triage doctor in labor and delivery examined her uterus with ultrasound and found a nine-centimeter blood clot in the uterus, near the placenta. The doctor was concerned that the placenta had partially abrupted or torn away from the wall of the uterus. He measured the amniotic fluid to be sure that none had leaked out and noted that the placenta appeared to have stopped separating from the uterus. After checking her thoroughly, he told Ann that she would have to stay in the hospital until they could be sure her bleeding had stopped and that she and her baby were stable. After a few days without further bleeding, her baby seemed to be doing fine, and an ultrasound confirmed there was no more abruption. She was told she could go home. Her obstetrician told her to maintain complete bed rest and sent a visiting nurse to do a fetal monitor test every few days for a while.

Ann was devastated and scared. She felt physically fine, but was told to stay in bed as much as possible. She called all her friends, who gladly helped her with errands, alleviating the boredom and helping Rick cope with the sudden change in their lives. Ann remained on modified bed rest with medication until the thirty-sixth week, nine weeks in all, but delivered Emma, her healthy eight-pound daughter at 37 weeks.

Ectopic Pregnancy

As you may remember from Chapter 2, when an embryo remains in a fallopian tube instead of implanting in the lining of the uterus—as it should—the pregnancy cannot continue. If left in place, the growing embryo will expand beyond the width of the fallopian tube and cause the tube to rupture.

Symptoms of ectopic pregnancy include bleeding early in the pregnancy and severe abdominal or shoulder pain. A suspected ectopic pregnancy is confirmed with ultrasound and a blood test that measures the level of the hormone human chorionic gonadotropin (hCG). This condition requires medical treatment to remove the embryo, either using medication or surgery.

Molar Pregnancy

If abnormal tissue develops from the fertilized egg instead of an embryo, the pregnancy will not develop into a baby. In some molar pregnancies there is a malformed embryo, and in others there's only abnormal tissue. Molar pregnancies are very rare.

The signs include vaginal bleeding in the first trimester, an abnormally large uterus, or swollen ovaries, and, in some cases, significantly elevated blood pressure. As with ectopic pregnancy, a molar pregnancy is diagnosed with a blood test that measures human chorionic gonadotropin (hCG), and it must be removed as well. Repeated hCG testing in the following six months will determine if any of the mole remains. Once hCG levels return to normal, talk with your OB provider about when you can try to become pregnant again.

Miscarriage

You may become pregnant but lose the fetus long before it can survive outside the womb. The loss of the fetus is called a *miscarriage*. Many miscarriages occur before women are even aware that they're pregnant. The March of Dimes states that between 15 and 20 percent of pregnancies end in miscarriage.[10]

Most miscarriages occur in the first trimester, before the twelfth week of pregnancy, and most occur because of problems in the development of the fetus. Women over 35 are more likely to have miscarriages than younger women. Most women who experience miscarriage are able to become pregnant again and have normal pregnancies.

The Stages of a Miscarriage

There are not different kinds of miscarriage, but there are different stages at which a miscarriage may occur. You may hear the following terms if you're having problems that could lead to the loss of your pregnancy:

- **Spontaneous abortion.** This is the medical term for a miscarriage. *Spontaneous*, of course, means "without warning," and to *abort* means "to bring forth." Therefore, a miscarriage is your body spontaneously bringing forth, or expelling, the pregnancy. (In medical terminology, a pregnancy that is ended electively is called a *voluntary termination of pregnancy*.)
- **Threatened miscarriage.** This refers to the early symptoms of miscarriage, such as spotting, bleeding, and cramping. About one in five women see some spotting in the first few weeks or months of being pregnant. This may be the beginning of a miscarriage, or it may merely be the shedding of a small amount of the uterine lining when the fertilized egg implants in the tissue of the uterus. Spotting can also occur from an irritation of the cervix during intercourse, or it can be the result of an infection. Your OB provider will try to determine the cause of your bleeding and tell you what to watch for, such as a significant increase in bleeding, blood clots, or cramping.
- **"Incomplete" miscarriage.** This means that not all of this material has been shed, and it may have to be removed by the doctor.
- **"Missed" miscarriage.** This type of miscarriage has no signs of shedding of the uterine lining—no spotting or bleeding—but when you're checked by ultrasound, your OB provider either finds an empty sac with no signs of a fetus or a fetus without signs of life.

Symptoms of Miscarriage

Symptoms of miscarriage include the following:

- **Spotting or bleeding from the vagina.** This may be as little as a small amount of spotting or as much as the heavy flow of menstrual bleeding. There may be blood clots. If you have bleeding, try to save a sample of the flow, particularly any solid material. Your doctor will have this material analyzed to confirm the miscarriage and to understand why a miscarriage has occurred.
- **Cramping, abdominal pain, or a feeling of pressure in the abdomen.** It may feel like gas pains or as if your stomach is upset from something you ate. The pain may either be sharp or dull, occasional or constant. Some women describe this early symptom as feeling like the start of a menstrual period.
- **Diminishment of morning sickness and fatigue.** With a missed miscarriage, your only clue may be that these usual symptoms of early pregnancy go away.

What Causes Miscarriage?

There are several discoverable causes of miscarriages, but, as noted above, in most cases the cause of the miscarriage is never found. First trimester miscarriages are more common, but the causes are not as detectable.

Causes of Early or First Trimester Miscarriages. These seem to occur most often when:

- *There are genetic defects in the embryo.* The cells of a spontaneously aborted fetus may reveal abnormalities in the chromosomes. Having a chromosomal abnormality may cause the embryo not to develop.
- *There's an imbalance in your hormones.* If not enough progesterone is produced, the lining of your uterus does not develop and cannot hold the growing embryo.
- *Your immune system is rejecting the baby.* Your body may be creating antibodies that attack your body's tissue. This is an *autoimmune disease.* A buildup of antibodies can be a problem for the fetus. One kind of antibody, *anticardiolipin*, makes blood clots

that disrupt the function of the placenta, which stops the fetus from receiving nutrients. Research is continuing into autoimmune disease and pregnancy.

- *Infections* in the genital tract are present that prevent all the components of fertilization and implantation.
- Specific things that may cause congenital problems with the embryo such as exposure to *environmental toxins*, smoking, taking drugs, or drinking alcohol, and chronic *medical conditions*, such as congenital heart disease, severe kidney disease, or uncontrolled diabetes.

Causes of Second Trimester Miscarriages. These are primarily caused by:

- An *abnormally shaped uterus*, called *congenital uterine malformation*.
- An *incompetent cervix*. Your cervix may not be strong enough to hold the enlarging fetus inside the uterus, and the cervix opens prematurely. See the section on incompetent cervix earlier in this chapter.
- *Uterine fibroids*. The hormones that stimulate pregnancy can also stimulate fibroids to grow. By the second trimester the fibroids are large enough to interfere with fetus growth. See the section on uterine fibroids in this chapter.
- *Preterm premature rupture of membranes (PPROM)*. When the membranes or bag of water surrounding the fetus breaks one hour before the onset of labor, this is a "preterm rupture of membranes" (PROM). When this rupture occurs in a mother who is less than 37 weeks gestation and one hour prior to labor, this is a "preterm premature rupture of membranes" (PPROM). When this occurs very early in the pregnancy, there are two possible outcomes. If the opening in the membrane seals over, preterm labor ceases, and sufficient fluid remains to sustain the fetus, the pregnancy continues. If an infection develops in the remaining fluid, preterm labor will ensue, and you may deliver an infant that cannot survive. Usually babies less than 22 weeks gestation cannot survive outside the womb.

Is Miscarriage Preventable?

Preventing a miscarriage is very difficult. There is no medication to stop it from happening once the fetus and placenta have begun to separate from the uterine lining.

If a miscarriage is threatening in the first trimester, your doctor or midwife will attempt to determine the cause of bleeding or spotting by:

- Carefully reviewing your medical history to determine if you have any medical conditions that could cause miscarriage.
- Checking your blood for signs of infection or an autoimmune disease.
- Performing a sonogram to determine whether the embryo is in the uterus or in a fallopian tube. If the fetus is in your uterus, the OB Provider will check to see if it has a heartbeat and is growing according to your due date.
- Checking to see that your cervix remains closed.
- Draw your blood to see, whether your pregnancy hormones are rising appropriately. This will confirm that your pregnancy is in the uterus versus a fallopian tube.
- Possibly asking you to increase rest and to stop having intercourse until the bleeding is resolved.
- Giving you hormone supplements if not enough progesterone is being produced.

If a miscarriage threatens in the second trimester, your doctor or midwife will use ultrasound to determine whether:

- The placenta is implanted improperly in the lining of your uterus.
- You have uterine fibroids.
- The fetus is growing abnormally.
- You have an abnormally shaped uterus or cervix.
- Your cervix is starting to thin out or open up.
- You need a cerclage.

With a threatened miscarriage in the second trimester, your doctor will probably ask you to rest and stay away from work for a while to see if your body can maintain the pregnancy. You'll be instructed to call if, your bleeding increases, you have cramping or abdominal pain, fever, blood clots, or heavy vaginal discharge.

How Is a Miscarriage Managed?

If you've lost the pregnancy, your doctor will use ultrasound to determine if all the tissues of the pregnancy—the fetus, placenta, and sac—have been expelled from your body. It's important to have any remaining material removed to avoid complications such as hemorrhaging or a severe infection. This material can be removed during a hospital or doctor's office visit with a procedure called a *suction dilatation and curettage* (D&C).

You'll feel cramping during the procedure, and sometimes, sharp pain. You may be given analgesics to relieve this pain. Sometimes some of the extracted material may be sent to the lab to see if it reveals the cause of your miscarriage.

After the D&C you'll be sent home with instructions to watch for excessive bleeding (more than one pad per hour), large blood clots (fist size), or signs of infection (fever, chills, and abdominal pain). Most women have no ongoing problems from the miscarriage, and after waiting the prescribed amount of time, can consider becoming pregnant again.

Emotional Recovery from a Miscarriage

Immediately after a miscarriage, you will probably be primarily concerned with how you are feeling physically. You will feel sore and may be very tired. After taking something for your discomfort and getting some sleep, what has happened will begin to sink in. You have lost your pregnancy, your plans for a baby. You may feel angry that nothing could be done to avoid this outcome. After anger, often comes guilt. You may dwell upon what you think you could or would have done to prevent this loss. You will question your decisions and your actions. "If only I would have taken more time to rest," "I wish I hadn't kept working so hard," "I shouldn't have had sex the night before," "I wanted this to happen because I didn't want to get pregnant in the first place." You may move back and forth between grief, anger, and guilt for several months.

While you are in the emotional recovery period, some days you may want to talk with family and friends or coworkers about your sadness. On other days you may want to pretend it didn't happen. Your family and friends may be tentative about approaching you or unsure about how to comfort you. They may try to tell you that you can always have another child or that the loss was for the best. This is probably not what you want to hear, but at first almost nothing they say will make you feel better.

There are several ways you can help yourself through this difficult time. You may find some comfort in having a keepsake of the pregnancy, perhaps an early sonogram or a baby toy. When you feel emotionally healed, you will be able to put this memento away. You can find a group of women who have had a similar experience. There are miscarriage support groups in most communities. You may find people you can talk to about how you are feeling within one of these groups. Ask your doctor about local groups or check on the Internet. There are also several national organizations that offer support. If you find yourself getting very depressed, unable to eat or sleep, and crying constantly, you may want to seek professional counseling and medication. While some women maintain that they never fully get over their miscarriages, most report that with the support of friends and family and, for some, with professional counseling, they are able to accept what has happened and move on with their lives.

Getting Pregnant Again After Miscarriage

Physically, your body will recover in a matter of weeks, but most doctors recommend their patients wait to try conceiving for four to six months. This allows your body to have a few normal menstrual cycles before starting a pregnancy. Your doctor may recommend a longer wait to have you undergo tests that could help determine the cause of your miscarriage.

The complications that can occur with pregnancy may mean some detours on your pregnancy journey, but with medical help they do not necessarily mean the journey will end early or badly. Try to think of these detours as an opportunity to learn more about your body and how it works, and how best to care for it, so that you complete your pregnancy journey with a healthy baby.

12

Thinking About Having
Another Child

 Barbara's Journal

> *Dear Journal,*
> *The time passed so quickly, I forgot about the morning sick-ness, the leg cramps, needing maternity clothes, the frequent interruptions during the night to go to the bathroom, and, toward the end, not being able to see my feet. So I'm thinking of having another child. I hope it will be better this time. I want to take better care of myself and be better prepared this time around.*

You and your partner are thinking about having another child. You feel you're ready for another pregnancy. There are a few things you may want to consider when starting to think about adding another baby to your family. Along with Chapter 1, this chapter will help you take stock of mental, physical, financial, and social factors that may be altered by a pregnancy and the addition of another child.

Planning to have another baby is a very personal and emotional choice. Answering the "What's Involved" questions following may help you decide if you're ready. Ask your partner to also think about the considerations raised by the questions.

Keep in mind that there is **no** *perfect time to have a baby, but you can plan wisely for the best future possible for everyone involved.*

What's Involved

Finances

- Do you have the finances to support another pregnancy and another child?
- Who is going to be the main financial provider?
- How will you pay for additional day care, health insurance, room in your house, baby equipment (if your older child is still using it), and baby supplies like diapers, food, formula, and so on.

Time

- If you may feel your time with your baby is limited now, how will you feel when you have to divide it further, to give some to another child?
- How will you take care of your child, get rest for yourself during your pregnancy, and work, either in the home or at a paying job?
- How do you feel about the amount and quality of time you have alone, and with your partner, now? Are there sufficient funds to pay for babysitting to give you more time together?

Your Health

- How did you like being pregnant before?
- Did you have an easy pregnancy?
- Do you feel like you've recovered?
- Do you feel ready to be pregnant again?
- Do you feel physically healthy, strong?
- Do you feel mentally or emotionally strong?
- Is your biological clock ticking?
- Did you have any difficulty getting pregnant before?
- Did you have any complications of pregnancy?
- Do you feel you have the support you need from your partner, family, and friends?

Your Baby's Health

- Did you have a healthy baby?
- Did you have a premature baby?
- Is your baby healthy now?

The Pros and Cons

The decision to have another child may depend upon your perceived ability to afford the costs of raising another child. Or one or both of you may feel that you already lack enough time for yourself and with each other, or lack time for your existing children. You may be reluctant to try for more than one or may decide to stop at two. Or you may have had complications in the earlier pregnancy, or your newest baby might have health problems. Or you're fearful of going through another physical and emotional trial.

The desire for a bigger family can override concerns about finances. Managing a household with two babies or more may seem more doable since you already have some idea of the impact on your time and money. Having had a difficult pregnancy or having a baby with health problems is often the biggest barrier to deciding to have another child. Fortunately, medical researchers are working hard to address complications of pregnancy, preterm labor, and premature birth.

Ongoing Medical Research

Medical science is trying to find clues to solving the mysteries of birth, labor, and preterm labor so that all newborn babies can receive the incomparable advantage of growing to full term in the womb. When every day can make a difference in the survival and health of a newborn baby, this research promises to halt or slow the steadily rising percentage of babies born prematurely. Most experts agree that despite all the medical advances for premature babies, the best incubator for a baby is still its mother's womb.

The areas of medical research currently under study fall into the following categories:

- *Identification* of those likely to have preterm labor
- *Development of new drugs* to prevent preterm labor
- *Research into new treatments* that can improve the health and survival rate of premature babies

Identification of Preterm Labor

Being able to accurately predict that a pregnant woman will deliver before full term—37 weeks gestation—would help ensure that both mother and baby get preventive preterm labor treatment as soon as possible. Currently, one of the strongest predictors of preterm labor and premature birth is a previous premature birth. Scientists and health care professionals would like to be able to better predict when preterm labor is likely to occur in women who have not previously given birth to a premature baby.

Studies are being conducted to learn more about what causes labor, and particularly preterm labor. If this mystery can be solved, scientists can work on discovering methods of predicting and preventing preterm delivery.

Development of New Drugs

Medications for women at risk for a premature delivery are also under scrutiny. Drug research is focusing on the development of more effective medications, more efficient delivery of these medications, and finding ways to reduce or eliminate adverse side effects.

Research into New Treatments

Finally, improving a premature baby's chances for survival and good health is the focus of many studies. Much of the current research focuses on improving treatment for premature babies' lungs. Other areas of study include improving care of premature babies' eyesight, brains, and digestive tracts.

From these three areas of study there will no doubt be tests and treatments available in the future that we can't even imagine right now. We mention these avenues of research in the hopes that if you're facing a high-risk pregnancy, you'll do your own research and become well informed about your options for protecting your own health and the health of all your babies—those already here and those you hope to have.

Knowledge is your best tool toward a healthy pregnancy and birth.

Committing to Another Baby After a Preemie

The decision to have another baby is difficult even in families with healthy, full-term babies. But if you've had a premature baby, you have a 17 to 37 percent chance of having another preterm birth.[1] With these odds, the difficulty of the decision increases exponentially.

If preterm labor recurs, bed rest and medication will be much more difficult while caring for your young child. In all likelihood, someone else will need to care for your child while you are on bed rest. You may also have ongoing concerns for the health of your first child. Premature babies often need extra medical care until they are two years old, and longer if there are continuing health problems. If your next baby is born prematurely, it will also need special care in the hospital and at home. You'll need to make arrangements for the care of your older child to be able to spend time with the newest one. This information is not to deter you but to give you points to consider when making your choice. Many couples with a premature baby go on to have other children and manage fairly well. After considering all the information, you will be better able to decide what is best for all of you.

Repeating Preconceptual Counseling

One final note: If you decide to try for another pregnancy, regardless of whether your previous pregnancy was high risk, you should check with your doctor to see if you should have preconceptual counseling again. Even though you'll feel like an "old hand" at pregnancy, it's important to have a thorough health evaluation before becoming pregnant.

Your doctor or midwife will be able to spot changes in your health profile since your last pregnancy. If you're having any problems that might make the next pregnancy difficult, such as infections or a chronic condition, these can be addressed or treated before you become pregnant. Your OB provider can also suggest beneficial changes to your diet and level of exercise so you start your pregnancy at a good weight and in good health.

Having been through pregnancy before, you have ample evidence of the importance of these preliminary preparations and you'll want to make your next pregnancy journey even better.

We hope this book has provided you and your partner with information that makes all your pregnancy journeys safer and smoother. You now have the tools to plan your journeys, and be confident that you'll be able to make the best decisions for your family. Once again, we wish you *bon voyage*!

Notes

Chapter 1

1. Joyce A. Martin et al., "Births: Final Data for 2001," *CDC National Vital Statistics Reports*, Dec. 18, 2002, 51(2):16.
2. Ibid.
3. "Doulas Ease Patient Labor," *American Academy of Family Physicians FP Report*, March 1998. This report cites 1996 research at Mount Sinai School of Medicine that when doulas were present, labor was shortened by 2.8 hours. It also cites a 1997 University of California–San Francisco study showing reduction in labor, fewer medications, and fewer cesareans. And it notes that a 1991 study cited by the *Journal of the American Medical Association* said that "in 412 women, rate of cesareans, epidurals, and forceps deliveries in 212 [were] less than half than in the control group of 200 women."

    "St. Vincent Hospital Initiates First Doula Program in New Mexico," Santa Fe Regional Medical Center, St. Vincent Hospital, Oct. 28, 1999. This report says, "Research has shown . . . having doulas decreases the rate of cesareans by 50 percent . . . and the length of labor by 25 percent."

    "Doula Services," Albert Einstein Healthcare Network, Jefferson Health System, says: "According to *Mothering the Mother*, a book written in 1993 by Klaus, Kennel, and Klaus, the presence of a doula shortens labor by an average of two hours, decreases cesareans by over 50 percent, and decreases the need for pain medication."

Chapter 2

1. "Age and Fertility, a Guide for Patients," American Society for Reproductive Medicine, 1996, 3; "Evaluating Infertility," ACOG Patient Education brochure, Washington, D.C., June 2000.
2. "Fertility, Family Planning, and Women's Health," CDC National Center for Health Statistics, Division of Data Services, June 26, 2001; "Evaluating Infertility," ibid.
3. "Infertility: An Overview, a Guide for Patients," American Society for Reproductive Medicine, 1995, 3.
4. "Age and Fertility, A Guide for Patients," American Society for Reproductive Medicine, 1996, 4.

5. Ibid, 8.
6. "Infertility: An Overview," 5.
7. "Facts About Endometriosis," National Institute of Child Health and Human Development, NIH publication 91-2413.
8. "Uterine Fibroids, a Guide for Patients," American Society for Reproductive Medicine, 1997, 5.
9. MEDLINEplus, U.S. National Library and the National Institute. "Semen Analysis," page 2.

Chapter 4

1. Joyce A. Martin, et al., "Births: Final Data for 2001," CDC *National Vital Statistics Reports*, Dec. 18, 2002, 51(2), 2002, 17; "Management of Preterm Labor Summary," *Evidence Report/Technology Assessment*, no. 18, Agency for Healthcare Research and Quality (AHRQ), Dec. 18, 2002.
2. UCI Medical Center, "March of Dimes Highlights Prematurity Campaign with Legislative Tour of UCI's Neonatal Intensive Care Unit," *March of Dimes Public Policy Research Report*, Aug. 14, 2003. The report quotes Manuel Porto, M.D.
3. Martin, ibid.
4. Lisa Potetz, "Request for Proposals: Public Health Insurance Programs and Preterm Birth." *March of Dimes Public Policy Research Report*, Oct. 2002; Martin, ibid, 18.
5. Joyce A. Martin and Melissa Park, "Trends in Twin and Triplet Births: 1980–97," CDC *National Vital Statistics Reports*, Sept. 1999, 47(24), 2; "Higher Order Multiple Births Drop for First Time in a Decade," National Center for Health Statistics, press release, April 17, 2001.
6. T. J. Mathews, MS., et al, "National Vital Statistics Reports Infant Mortality Statistics from the 2000 Period Linked Birth/Infant Death Data Set," CDC *Monthly Vital Statistics Report*, Aug. 28, 2002, 50(12), 7; "New CDC Data Show Preterm Births Down Among African Americans," News Release, CDC Division of Media Relations, March 11, 1999.
7. Potetz, ibid.
8. *High Risk Clinical Conditions in Pregnancy—A Case Management Reference Manual*, Tokos Clinical Services Corporation, 1993, page 49.
9. *Having Twins*, ACOG Patient Education brochure, Washington, D.C., Sept. 1998.
10. Stephanie J. Ventura and Joyce Martin, "Advance Report of Final Natality Statistics," CDC *Monthly Vital Statistics Report*, Sept. 9, 1993, 42/3: 7, 13.

Chapter 6

1. Mary Hammond-Tooke, "Predicting Preterm Labor," *Maternity Center Special Delivery*, Spring 2000, 1; R. P. Heine et al., "Serial Salivary Estriol to Detect an Increased Risk of Preterm Birth," *Obstetrics and Gynecology*,

PubMed, National Library of Medicine (Internet), Oct. 2000, 96(4): 490–497.

Chapter 7

1. Work Group on Breastfeeding, Lawrence M. Gartner, MD, Chairperson, et al. "Breastfeeding and the Use of Human Milk (RE-9729)," *American Academy of Pediatrics Policy Statement*, Dec. 1997, 100(6): 1035–1039.
2. Ibid, 1038.
3. Joyce A. Martin et al., "Births: Final Data for 2001," *CDC National Vital Statistics Reports*, Dec. 18, 2002, 51(2), 77, Table 42.

Chapter 8

1. *Postpartum Depression*, ACOG Patient Education brochure, Washington, D.C., March 1999.
2. "Trends in Unintended Pregnancy," *The Contraception Report, Contraception Online: Contraception and Reproductive Health Info of OB/GYN Professionals*, May 1998, page 3. Cites S. K. Henshaw, "Unintended Pregnancy in the United States." *Family Planning Perspective* 1998;30:24–29, 46.

Chapter 10

1. Joyce A. Martin and Melissa M. Park, "Trends in Twin and Triplet Births: 1980–97," *CDC National Vital Statistics Reports*, vol. 47, no. 24, Sept. 1999, 2.
2. Ibid, 3.
3. Ibid, 2.
4. Ibid, 8–9.
5. Gary F. Cunningham, M.D., et al. *William's Obstetrics* (20th edition). Appleton and Lang; Simon & Schuster, 1997, 864.
6. "Having Twins," ACOG Patient Education brochure, Washington, D.C., Sept. 1998.
7. Martin and Park,"Trends in Twin and Triplet Births: 1980–97," 4.
8. Ibid.

Chapter 11

1. The National Cancer Institute, National Institute of Child Health and Human Development, National Institutes of Health. "Women Who Took DES, A Guide of Women Who Took DES During Pregnancy From 1938 to 1971," DES Publications, National DES Education Program, September 1993.
2. "Uterine Fibroids," American Society for Reproductive Medicine, 1997.
3. Gary F. Cunningham, M.D., et al. *William's Obstetrics* (20th edition). Appleton and Lange; Simon & Schuster, 1997, page 306.
4. "Group B Strep Infection," March of Dimes Health Library Fact Sheets, 2002.

5. Ibid.
6. "Tracking the Hidden Epidemics, Trends in STDs in the United States, 2000," CDC. Page 24. cdc.gov/nchstp/dstd/Stats_Trends/Trends2000.pfd; Gary F. Cunningham, et al. *Williams' Obstetrics*, 20th ed. Appleton & Lange; Simon & Schuster, 1997, pages 312–313.
7. "Bleeding During Pregnancy," ACOG Patient Education brochure, Washington, D.C., April 1999.
8. Gary F. Cunningham, M.D., et al. *William's Obstetrics* (20th edition). Appleton and Lange; Simon & Schuster, 1997, page 1206.
9. Joyce A. Martin et al., "Births: Final Data for 2001," CDC *National Vital Statistics Reports*, Dec. 18, 2002, 51(2), 77, Table 42.
10. "Miscarriage," March of Dimes Health Library Fact Sheets, 2000, www.mod-imes.org/HealthLibrary/.

Chapter 12

1. David G. Weismiller, M.D., SC.M., "Preterm Labor," American Family Physician, American Academy of Family Physicians, February 1999. page 2. cites for these statistics from the American College of Obstetricians and Gynecologists. "Preterm Labor. Committee opinion no. 206. Washington, D.C.: ACOG, 1995.

Index

Eating habits, 9, 52
Ectopic pregnancy, 81, 274
Effacement, 131–132, 169
Egg cells, 43–46, 51, 55, 56–57, 63–64
Ejaculation problems, 61–62
Electrolytes, 135, 171
Embryo, 45, 82
Endocrine system, 52
Endometrial biopsy, 54
Endometriosis, 58–59
Endometrium, 45, 48–49, 54, 60
Enemas, 171
Engorgement, 191
Epidural block, 29, 31, 34, 92, 161–162, 180, 189
Epilepsy, 7
Episiotomy, 177, 188
Estriol, 133
Estrogen, 44, 55, 57, 59, 78, 254
Ethylene glycol, 22
Exercise:
  during bed rest/activity reduction, 225–227
  diabetes and, 270, 271
  fertility and, 52
  postpartum, 194, 198–201
  in preconceptual planning, 19, 26
  before pregnancy, 9, 10–12
  during pregnancy, 74–76, 83–84, 89–91, 92–93, 95, 153
  safety measures for, 12, 75–76
  in stress reduction, 17
External cephalic version, 167

Failure to progress, 162, 179–180, 182–183
Fallopian tubes, 43–44, 59, 60, 81, 274
False labor, 120–121, 168
Family Leave Act, 215
Family medical history, 23–24
Fat substitutes, 73
Fatigue, 77–78, 95, 193, 194, 196, 202, 276
Fats, 13, 15, 69, 70, 71, 79
FDA (Food and Drug Administration), 8–9, 27, 108
Fears, 39–40, 65, 84
Ferning, 133
Fertility calendar, 47
Fertility. *See* Infertility
Fertilization, 43–49
Fetal alcohol syndrome (FAS), 107–108
Fetal development, 7–8, 82–98. *See also* Assessment of fetus
Fetal distress, 180
Fetal fibronectin, 132–133
Fetal heart monitor, 118, 129–130, 135, 141, 172, 180, 240
Fetoscope, 173, 233–234
Fiber, 13, 69, 72, 95, 192–193
Fibroids, 59–60, 105, 255, 265, 277

Fibronectin, 132–133
Filipinos, 24
First trimester, 76–84
Flagyl, 259
Flu, 20
Folic acid, 13, 14, 26–27, 42, 241
Follicular-stimulating hormone (FSH), 44, 45, 55, 56, 57
Food and Drug Administration (FDA), 8–9, 27, 108
Food cravings, 80–81
Forceps delivery/extraction, 163, 177–178
Fragile X, 23, 25
Fruits, 13–14, 70, 71, 72
Full-term birth, 165
Fundal height, 233
Fundal massage, 185–186
Fundus, 233

Gamma rays, 22
Gaslike pain, 116, 117, 119, 192, 193
General anesthesia, 163–164, 180, 181, 189
Genetic screening/testing, 23–25, 84
German measles (rubella), 20, 23
Ginger, 80
Glucocorticoids/glucocorticosteroids, 139, 140
Glucose tolerance test (GTT), 269–270
Gonadotropin (GTN), 56
Gonadotropin-releasing hormone (GnRH), 45, 56
Gonorrhea, 53, 59, 135
Grains, 13–14, 70, 72
Greeks, 24
Group B Beta streptococcus (GBS), 135, 257, 258–259

Harmful agents, 8–9, 20–26, 51–52, 62, 72–73, 107–110, 277
Headaches, 263
Health insurance coverage (*see* Insurance coverage)
Heart disease, 7
Heartburn, 95, 242
Hemoglobin, 267
Hemophilia, 23, 25
Hemorrhoids, 72, 192–193
Hepatitis A, 20
Hepatitis B, 20, 22, 136
Heroin, 108
High blood pressure, 7, 20, 68, 96, 105, 179, 262–264
Hispanics, 269
HMOs (Health Maintenance Organizations), 30–31
Home contraction monitors, 246
Home delivery, 30–31, 33–34
Home pregnancy tests, 49

About the Authors

Bonnie C. Campos is currently the Director of Women's Health Services at Kaiser Permanente Mid-Atlantic States Region. She has worked in the field of high-risk obstetrics with various programs in Colorado, Maryland, Virginia, and the District of Columbia.

She received her bachelor of science degree in nursing from the University of Colorado Health Sciences Center and completed a master of science degree in women's health at the University of Maryland, Baltimore. She is certified as an OB/GYN Nurse Practitioner.

She developed an award-winning Premature Prevention Program called TLC or Tender Loving Care for Kaiser Permanente in 1990. Her primary focus is to oversee current programs within Kaiser Permanente that address contemporary issues of women's health.

Jennifer C. Brown is a writer who also works in film and video production. She specializes in health and safety subjects. She has a bachelor of arts degree in art from Allegheny College in Pennsylvania and a master of art degree in communications from American University. She lives in Silver Spring, Maryland, with her husband and two sons.